WHY IS AMERICA SO SICK?

LINKING DIGESTIVE HEALTH TO IMMUNITY AND HORMONAL ISSUES

JOANNE M. CONAWAY, BSN, RN, ND

FOREWORD BY JONATHAN W. EMORD

Why Is America So Sick?

ISBN: 978-1-943157-03-7

Printed in the United States of America

For more information or how to reach Dr. Joanne Conaway, go to:

www.DrJConaway.com

WHAT OTHERS ARE SAYING

I have been on nutritional products for the past 13 years and have seen many benefits but continued to struggle with extreme digestion issues; stomach problems and constipation my whole life. I learned all my issues came from poor absorption and an unhealthy digestive system. I had fibromyalgia and my doctor said I would be crippled in a few years and unable to work. Other issues were arthritis, carpal tunnel from house cleaning, rashes all over my body, severe itchy skin that often broke in hives, hair falling out, and fatigue.

I went to a meeting where I met Dr. Joanne Conaway. She was talking about different conditions that result from poor absorption and an unhealthy gut. I was in every category she talked about. I followed her protocol closely and have been amazed at the results. With the enzymes, probiotics and proper nutrition that she talks about, my body is normalizing in ways I was told from the medical profession I never would. I never go without my flora and enzymes. Thank you Dr. Conaway!!

—V.W., Riverton, UT

I have suffered from tummy issues all of my life. As a five-year-old girl, medical doctors began running tests to try and determine why I had stomach aches all the time. When they could not find a cause they attributed it to stress. Really? I was five!

As I grew up, I learned to live with the discomforts and even began to assume that everyone else felt the same way as I did. It was my normal. About a year ago, I learned from Dr. Conaway that I could easily address the pain, bloating, and discomfort. With hope I applied her protocol and within days I began to feel the difference.

By the time I completed the protocol, the intestinal problems I had lived with all of my life were erased. For the first time I knew what it was like to NOT have pain! Now whenever I have discomfort I know that something is "off" and I return to her simple protocol. Problem solved! I can't thank her enough!

—K.H., Mesa, AZ

Dr. Conaway is so knowledgeable but more importantly than that, she is an attentive listener and genuinely cares. After struggling with digestion and other health obstacles since I was 15, my mom and I have searched for solutions. As the years went on I began to feel hopeless. Working with Dr. Conaway has allowed me to believe I can once again find my optimal health. For that I cannot thank her enough.

—M. S., Scottsdale, AZ

ACKNOWLEDGMENTS

Any good author will tell you a job like writing a book is not as simple as putting the words on paper. In the case of this book, I have several people to thank.

First, my husband, Rich, my biggest devotee, who has encouraged me every step of the way. He was always there and would stop whatever he was doing to listen, to offer suggestions, and to help wordsmith when my brain considered it time to take a break. This may not have been completed and certainly not in a timely fashion, had it not been for his willingness to do whatever it took to keep the home fires burning. I am so lucky to have him and his endless support.

Also, it takes hours to write a book but many more hours to ensure punctuation and spelling are correct. My sincere appreciation for all the time, effort, and reassurance as I accomplished this task goes to my good friend, Phyllis Anderson. She gave up weekends and often worked into the night to help me bring this to completion. Her suggestions, corrections, recommendations, and well-trained eye certainly enhanced the finished product.

To Dr. Joel Wallach. A special thank you for his mentorship and for introducing me to an approach to lasting health and wellness I can get excited about. He helped me recognize and understand the rewards of sharing his powerful message and I will be forever grateful.

Lastly, to my many friends and supporters. You know who you are and I thank you for all the prayers and encouragement as I worked to bring this to completion.

DEDICATION

To my loving husband, Richard, who has provided endless support and encouragement over the years, as I pursued my education, change of career, and most recently in the production of this book. There are no words to express my gratitude for all the time he put into my endeavor. Thank you, sweetheart.

To my son, Richard ("Rhett"), whose personal experiences fueled my passion for the study, and sharing, of this message.

To Blake Graham, a friend and true supporter who stood by my decision to pursue this endeavor, mentored me, and who is in fact the person responsible for the title of this book. Blake's friendship and support helped me realize my goals and I will be forever grateful.

FOREWORD

Few people educated in conventional medicine and care have the courage to challenge the very system that provides them with income and employment. There are few willing to challenge fundamental precepts that underlie the medical establishment. Dr. Joanne Conaway is among the courageous few. Her military background in service to her country in the theater of war is but one proof of her uncommon courage. She has acquired a tremendous education concerning the hazards of drug dependency, not illicit drug dependency, but legal drug dependency. She knows well that when a medical paradigm that is designed for crisis intervention becomes one of common resort for a large and ever growing population of Americans, the chronic sickness that befalls this class of dependent people threatens the very fabric of American life.

We were not born to be patients and yet the conventional medical paradigm views each of us as dependents who will sooner or later rely on drug prescriptions for every ailment, possible symptom, or inconvenience. That approach leads to a sick and dependent culture, precisely the one Dr. Conaway finds befalling America today and the one she so eagerly seeks to eliminate.

The disease treatment paradigm accepted by conventional medical practitioners creates a crisis management mentality. Individuals receive the most health care not while healthy but when in dire straits, often after arriving at the emergency room suffering from a serious ailment. It is at that time when the individual is least able to fend for him or herself and is most willing to accept any medical recommendation in the hopes of recovery. It is at that time when individuals are most vulnerable to the foibles of modern medicine: to receipt of a wrong diagnosis, to receipt of a dangerous prescription drug, and to receipt of the wrong intervention. Rationality gives way to urgent need.

Moreover, the entire paradigm for medicine, from the local clinic to the FDA drug approval process depends on drug interventions for the treatment of disease and symptoms of disease. The approach often avoids a cure in favor of masking signs and symptoms of disease in the hope that the body will cure itself. While youthful patients can fare well with recovery, older ones do not ordinarily. While we depend on nutrients to repair and restore the body to normal, modern medicine views dietary supplementation and nutritional interventions with a jaundiced eye, albeit increasingly more conventional practitioners are coming to realize that they must embrace nutrition.

Dr. Joanne Conaway offers a different approach. Dr. Conaway recognizes that longevity is dependent upon healthy interventions that are best adopted when we are not in extremis but when we are still on our own two feet and that those interventions depend upon vigilant application throughout life. Dr. Conaway prescribes changes in diet and lifestyle, with a particular emphasis on gut health. She seeks to empower the individual to transform his or her own health without heavy reliance on crisis intervention from conventional medicine. She is not an enemy of conventional medicine, having been conventionally trained and experienced, but she is very definitely a friend of natural medicine. In particular, she wants to enable each of us, through education about wise food, supplementation, and lifestyle choices, to correct the dire course America now experiences through informed self-help.

As Dr. Conaway puts it, America is sick. Increasingly, our population suffers from chronic maladies as never before: diabetes, heart disease, cancer, respiratory illness, psychological illness, and digestive illnesses. We are indeed a nation of ill people, and we are also a nation of drug dependent people. Dr. Conaway wants to wean us of our dependency on drugs and revive us through a return to healthy, non-GMO foods; to supplementation that replenishes the lost vitamins and minerals from our depleted soils and, arising therefrom, food stocks; and to self-help, whereby we learn to take responsibility for our health so that we can avoid disease.

We will all experience medical crises in this life, but if we follow the path Dr. Conaway provides for us in this book, we are more apt to experience fewer crises and longer periods of wellness. Adhering to

Dr. Conaway's recommendations does require us to educate ourselves about disease, human biology, and the effects of foods and lifestyle on our risk of disease. It is well worth the investment in reading time and behavior change, however, because with greater knowledge, correct food and supplementation choices, and self-reliance, we can experience the extraordinary transformations in life that Dr. Conaway wants for us.

We can view the world through a healthy prism that enables us to avoid bad food choices, adopt healthy supplementation alternatives, and reduce reliance on conventional medicine, or we can continue on the wayward path now so common where we eat poorly, avoid nutritional interventions, and depend chronically on medical help. We can change a culture of sickness and medical dependency into one of wellness and independence if only we take heed to the wise approach Dr. Conaway recommends.

—Jonathan W. Emord

TABLE OF CONTENTS

INTRODUCTION

As I sit here preparing to put pen to paper, I find myself compelled to look back on the past 40 years or so that I have been involved in the medical field to consider where I started and where the journey has taken me. I must start out saying I am not against Western medicine. It has provided me numerous different job opportunities and a comfortable lifestyle.

To give you some idea of the type of person I am, it took me six years and three changes in major to finally choose nursing as a career. My mom was a nurse and that seemed like the best choice for me at the time. Graduating with a Bachelor's Degree in nursing in 1976, I began my journey as a professional. Through my school years I had worked as a nurses' aide starting in Pediatrics and then in the Emergency Room. Training at a major trauma and teaching hospital, Scott & White in Temple, Texas, I found the Emergency Room a very exciting and stimulating place to work. As fate would have it, there was not a job for me in the ER upon graduation and I instead started in the Intensive Care Unit. What an experience that turned out to be. I cared primarily for immediate post-op, open heart surgery patients, and the critical pediatric patients because of my prior experience and love of children. Caring for pediatric patients, especially those critically ill, was a challenge and forced me to mature quickly. The work was rewarding and certainly educational, working with all the interns, residents and a senior medical staff that included some of the best minds in medicine. I could not have received better training anywhere in the country. Little did I know then how much I would appreciate that amazing training later in life.

Never one to miss an opportunity to do something exciting, I spent only a few minutes getting to "Yes, that's a great idea" as my answer when my roommate came home one day and told me she thought it would be fun to talk with recruiters and see what opportunities there might be for the two of us in the military. I had been raised in a Navy household, so military life was something familiar and comfortable, and off we went. We found the most potentially exciting choices were those given us by the U.S. Air Force. Commissioned in August 1977, off I went on a new adventure. I spent three years on active duty, trained as an OR nurse, and finished my tour of duty back in the ICU. After those three years I went immediately into the Air Force Reserves, was trained as a Flight Nurse, and spent the next 13 years attached to the 34th Aeromedical Evacuation Squadron at Kelly Air Force Base in Texas. I flew around the country and the world training to be ready for the "call." I had the chance to answer that call in December 1989 as we deployed into Panama for "Operation Just Cause"; also in January 1991 to set up a staging facility in England during the first "Operation

Desert Storm." My reserve career and 20 years of service culminated at the U.S. Air Force Academy in Colorado Springs, Colorado, retiring as a Lt. Colonel after an amazing 20-year adventure.

During the 17 years of reserve duty I continued my civilian career as a nurse. I worked in several disciplines within nursing including Nursing Education and Infection Control, the OR, Recovery Room, Med/Surg, and Management. The area of most important impact that led me where I am today was my job as a Nutritional Support Nurse. My team consisted of two Nephrologists, myself, another RN, two Registered Dieticians, and a PhD Pharmacist. I was now back at Scott & White at a time when understanding and technology provided us the opportunity to nutritionally support patients who could no longer eat by mouth. We kept them alive with specialized tube feeding or intravenous formulations. We were all learning, spending time daily doing research and lab interpretation to determine the actual nutritional needs of the patients we monitored in the hospital and saw as outpatients in the clinic. Uncovering facts and recognizing the body needed more than just protein, carbohydrates, and fats to function properly, led to the addition of specific mineral and trace minerals to the formulas. We learned these were necessary to support the nutritional needs at the cellular level. This enlightening knowledge made me question why commercially prepared supplements did not include more of those minerals and trace minerals.

Busy with my careers (civilian and military), starting a family, and moving on to other nursing adventures, I lost focus and did not ponder the question for many years. Then in 1998 I received a copy of the cassette tape "Dead Doctors Don't Lie" by Dr. Joel D. Wallach, DVM, ND. I was struck by his very powerful message that revealed the understanding and proof that most chronic disease and illness are the result of a nutritional deficiency: more specifically in many cases, a mineral or trace mineral deficiency. That reignited a spark, and led me to research and re-learn as much as I could about the link between deficiencies and disease, leading ultimately to my desire to pursue a career as a naturopath.

I eagerly started exploring these new topics. I knew Dr. Wallach's message was right on due to my own experience observing the manifestations of deficiency diseases in the patients I worked with and cared for. I devoured all the information I could get my hands on. While doing so, I had the chance to observe firsthand, in my son, the impact of this healthy nutritional approach. With the addition of probiotics to his nutritional regimen we were able to correct his eight-year struggle with eczema in a matter of a few days. That transformation led me to a more in-depth study of how the digestive system plays a critical role in immunity, as well as how a healthy, supported digestive system could correct a chronic problem in just a few short days.

My passion for this subject is profound. What I have learned is, at least in part, shared on the following pages as I feel this is information everyone needs to maintain good health. My specific approach to the restoration of a healthy digestive system has helped people correct long-term problems, not only of skin issues like eczema, but chronic health issues like arthritis, autoimmune disorders, digestive issues like chronic constipation, irritable bowel syndrome, Crohn's disease, and so on. I am fond of saying I have helped more people in the last 16 years with superior nutritionals than I ever helped in almost 40 years of nursing.

WHY IS AMERICA SO SICK?

PART I

CHAPTER 1

SEEING THE BIG PICTURE

Your Health—Your Choice

What is health? It is defined as:

- The condition of being well or free from disease (*Merriam-Webster Dictionary*)
- The state of being free from illness/disease or injury/ailment
- The general condition of the body or mind with reference to soundness and vigor (Dictionary.reference.com)
- "A state of complete physical, mental, and social well-being and not merely the absence of disease and infirmity" ("Preamble," Constitution of the World Health Organization, 1946—remains controversial)[1]

These are all similar definitions. One might argue they are not complete as, more than ever, people are now considering body, mind and spirit as we define health.

What is choice? It is defined as:

- The act of selecting or making a decision when two or more choices are available (*Merriam-Webster Dictionary*)
- The power, right or liberty to choose (Dictionary.com)
- A range of possibilities from which one or more may be chosen (*Oxford Dictionary*)

Again, similar definitions, but let's think about health and choice together. I would say healthy choices would be those conducive to good health; choices indicative of sound, rational thinking or frame of mind and choosing a lifestyle that leaves you fit, energetic and at reduced risk for disease.

No matter how you might define healthy choice or put it into context for your life, the important thing to remember is *you are in control*. You have the right to make decisions you feel will benefit you from a health perspective. You have the choice to pick the kinds of foods you want to eat, the water you want to drink, the supplements you want to take, all the lifestyle choices that will lead you down the path of vibrant good health or its alternative; the path of dismal, ill health.

Having control and making "right" choices requires knowledge and understanding, therefore some education. Your control requires you to pay attention once you understand what is best, and often requires you to make tough choices. Who doesn't want that piece of chocolate cake or the second or third glass of wine? Pick your poison, if you will, and before making that impulsive decision consider what impact that decision will have on your good health.

It is not enough to simply want to make good choices. Making choices without education and knowledge can lead to serious consequences. I work with so many people who face chronic illness each day, making unhealthy choices, because they don't know what they don't know. Let's take a minute to look at some concerning statistics.

Statistics

Is America so sick? I think most would agree that each day we observe an increase in the numbers of people of all ages diagnosed with chronic degenerative diseases, cardiac diseases, neurological diseases, endocrine diseases, psychological diseases, and cancer.

Consider the following statistics. Many of these come from the CDC.gov website. The Centers for Disease Control and Prevention is one of the best bodies of number crunchers I know, working tirelessly to provide us with statistical data. Though they do not make laws that govern the health and wellness of this country, many of the laws we have, governing health care and standards of practice, come about based on their recommendations.

Autism
– 2012; 1 in 88 children, compared to 1 in 5,000 in the mid-1970s (CDC)

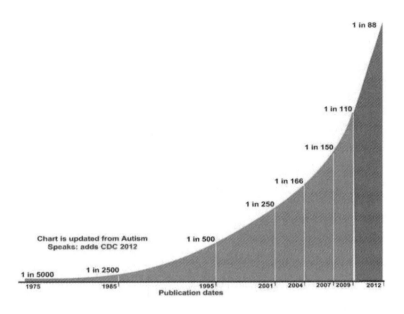

Figure 1 http://www.carinoga.com/wp-content/uploads/2014/03/rate-ride-autism.jpg

Currently the Centers for Disease Control and Prevention (CDC) estimates 1 in 68 children (or 14.7 per 1,000 eight-year-olds) in multiple communities in the United States has been identified with autism spectrum disorder (ASD). This new estimate is roughly 30 percent higher than previous estimates reported in 2012 of 1 in 88 children (11.3 per 1,000 eight-year-olds) being identified with an autism spectrum disorder. The number of children identified with ASD ranged from 1 in 175 children in Alabama to 1 in 45 children in New Jersey. The data continue to show that ASD is almost five times more common among boys than girls: 1 in 42 boys versus 1 in 189 girls. White children are more likely to be identified as having ASD than are black or Hispanic children.[2]

12

These numbers have increased significantly over the course of the last several years. The CDC has stated that:

> The recent prevalence increase [of ASD] is likely attributable to extrinsic factors such as improved awareness and recognition and changes in diagnostic practice or service availability.

> This is supported by the fact that recent statistics have noted an increase in the incidence of autism in specific populations and racial backgrounds, suggesting increasing awareness in such groups.

Researchers can't seem to agree on the real reason why the numbers have increased so dramatically. The possibilities given are that the definition has been expanded over the last several years, there is a heightened awareness surrounding the diagnosis, maybe an actual increase in the incidence, or some combination of all of these.

Making the diagnosis is not an exact science. We are now finding many children on the autism spectrum or diagnosed with autism spectrum disorder (ASC). Some feel the increase in numbers has more to do with the broadening of the diagnosis and expanding it to include other disorders, which fell outside the criteria for the spectrum disorder up until the new criteria were published in 2013. I am convinced it has more to do with the environment. Our food supply, the toxic soup we live in and the endless numbers of vaccinations must play a role.

ADD/ADHD
– March 2013; 1 in 10 (CDC)

The American Psychiatric Association states in the *Diagnostic and Statistical Manual of Mental Disorders* (DSM-5) that 5% of children have ADHD. Studies in the U.S. have estimated higher rates in community samples:

The percent of children estimated to have ADHD has also changed over time. Consider these statistics:

> Approximately 11% of children 4–17 years of age (6.4 million) have been diagnosed with ADHD as of 2011.

> The percentage of children with an ADHD diagnosis continues to increase, from 7.8% in 2003 to 9.5% in 2007 and to 11.0% in 2011.

> Rates of ADHD diagnosis increased an average of 3% per year from 1997 to 2006 and an average of approximately 5% per year from 2003 to 2011.

> Boys (13.2%) were more likely than girls (5.6%) to have ever been diagnosed with ADHD.

> The average age of ADHD diagnosis was 7 years of age, but children reported by their parents as having more severe ADHD were diagnosed earlier.

> Prevalence of ADHD diagnosis varied substantially by state, from a low of 5.6% in Nevada to a high of 18.7% in Kentucky.[3]

If those numbers don't make people sit up and take notice, we are in real trouble.

Type 2 Diabetes
– Rates in the U.S. increased by 176 percent between 1980 and 2011 (CDC)

From 1980 through 2011, the crude prevalence of diagnosed diabetes increased 176% (from 2.5% to 6.9%). During this period, increases in the crude and age-adjusted prevalence of diagnosed diabetes were similar, indicating that most of the increase in prevalence was not because of changes in the population age structure.[4]

Celiac Disease
– Now four times more common than 60 years ago

The prevalence of celiac disease is rising dramatically. Joseph Murray, M.D., a Mayo gastroenterologist, says celiac disease is becoming a public health issue. Studies show four times the incidence compared to 1950, with fatal complications if it goes untreated.

"Celiac disease was rare, but it's now more common in all age groups," Dr. Murray says. Although the cause is unknown, celiac disease affects about one in 100 people. What's more, Mayo has found a fourfold higher death risk for people with undiagnosed gluten intolerance.[5]

Alzheimer's Disease
– Rates have doubled since the 1980s, an alarming increase.

It is estimated that 5.2 million Americans (one in eight older Americans) had AD in 2014. It is the sixth leading cause of death and almost two-thirds of Americans with Alzheimer's disease are women.[6]

The following graph portrays how many Americans over the age of 65 are currently affected by Alzheimer's, as well as projecting how many more will be affected as time passes, according to The University of Oklahoma Health Sciences Center.

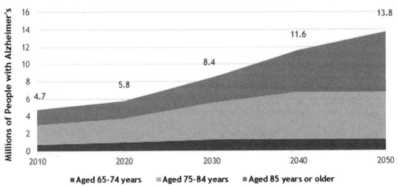

Figure 2 http://www.chicagoeb5.com/wp-content/uploads/2014/08/grafica12.jpg

Now, if you take a few minutes and ponder these numbers, really contemplate the dramatic increases, I think you'll have to agree America is so sick. Yes, you can spend days looking through all the research being done and the enormous impact this is having on health care. The charts and graphs are all there and the researchers are pointing to any number of reasons why we might be seeing these statistics skyrocket. But do they really have the answers?

It's All In Your Genes

I, for one, am hard pressed to believe many of these theories, especially the ones that are prompting extensive genetic research. Are researchers really trying to convince me we are unmasking a specific, formerly undetected, gene or gene sequence in all these people? Are all these newly diagnosed autism spectrum disorder patients born with a new or recently mutated gene? What about all the children with peanut allergies? Are they all born with a new or recently mutated gene? It just doesn't add up and does not make good scientific sense to me.

What it does do is create special research projects requiring billions in research grant money or government funding so we can find the "answer."

Gene Theories

Let's consider genes for a moment.

Scientists have long known that four bases— adenine (A), thymine (T), cytosine (C) and quinine (G)—make up the genetic code. These letters provide the recipes for proteins, which carry out numerous bodily functions. But there are still questions to be answered. How are the 3.2 billion base pairs contained in the human genome ordered? This is the person's entire bundle of DNA, divided evenly among 23 pairs of chromosomes. To that end, the Human Genome Project (HGP) was launched in 1990. Some of the project's ambitious goals included:

- Sequencing the entire human genome
- Identifying human genes
- Charting variations across human genomes
- Sequencing genomes of the mouse and four other "model organisms"

The project was run by the National Institutes of Health and the U.S. Department of Energy and completed ahead of schedule in 2003. Final results were published in 2006, but the data produced have since been continually examined, analyzed, and occasionally revised.

Some of what was learned surprised many, especially the scientists as they predicted that humans had up to 100,000 genes. Recent HGP estimates lowered that number to a more modest range of 20,000 to 25,000.[7] However, as of January 2014, it is reported the human genome shrinks to only 19,000. It turns out we had fewer genes than the nematode worm. "Our evidence suggests that the final number of true protein coding genes in the reference genome may lie closer to 19,000 then to 20,000."[8]

So the Human Genome Project, a massive $3 billion global effort dedicated to deciphering the human genetic code, is a failure? Many interesting facts have been revealed during the years following completion of the project. Bruce Lipton points out in *The Biology of Belief* the project was actually designed by venture capitalists, something I didn't suspect. These people figured that since there were over 100,000 genes, if the genes could be identified, and gene sequences patented, they could sell the gene patents to the drug industry. The drug industry would then use them to create health products and medicines specific to the gene sequence. The truth is, the program was not actually for advancing the human state as much as it was for making a lot of money.

It was thought the completed human blueprint would provide science with all the necessary information to "cure" all of mankind's ills. It was further assumed that an awareness of the human genetic code mechanism would enable scientists to create a Mozart or another Einstein.[9] Now that's a scary thought.

Since the human genome was sequenced, over 10 years ago, hardly a week has gone by without some new genetic "breakthrough" being reported. Each week new genes, for any number of diseases, generate sometimes front–page news across the globe.[10] People rush off to make an appointment to be tested. After all, that "X" gene might be the cause of their unusual symptoms. Once they know for sure, based on expensive testing (not often covered by health insurance), they may well be offered a prescription for the latest expensive drug (also not often paid for by insurance). This drug, developed to treat their symptoms, will make life better. Of course this puts more money into the pockets of the research facilities, the drug companies and, of course, the MDs as they must examine you (and charge for an office visit), order the test, then write the prescription.

Take a closer look and you'll find the reality is very different. Among all the genetic findings for common illnesses, such as heart disease, cancer and mental illnesses, only a handful are of genuine significance for human health. Research has learned faulty genes rarely cause, or even *mildly* predispose us to disease. Consequently, the science of human genetics is not what was hoped for. It is, in fact, a way for big medicine and big pharma to make billions each year. It is any wonder our health care system is in such a mess?

CHAPTER 2

CHOICES AND INFLUENCES

Food

We all need to eat. However, food today is simply not what it used to be.

When we look back historically at the food our ancestors ate, it was nothing like what we have in the food supply today. History will tell us various different things. There were times when food was very expensive. Depending on weather conditions, food was scarce, many times there was no meat available, and people survived on vegetables and healthy grains. For the most part in the late 19th and early 20th centuries, people ate what was grown locally and choices were limited. Sweets were a luxury. If it didn't come from your garden or you were not able to get it at the local market, you simply did not have it.

Most of us could not survive in a world like that. Consider what we have today. The majority of people live in or close to the city and there is always a grocery store just a few miles away. There is abundance, there is selection, and there is more than enough food for us to eat. It would seem that because we have ample amounts, we should all be healthy; at least not hungry. After all it's there, it's available, it's in the budget, and therefore I eat.

But what are we eating? Let's take a look at prepackaged and processed foods, for example. Without a doubt they are convenient, easy to prepare, and often substantial in providing that "full feeling"; but what are they really and are they good for us? If you look at the nutrition panel on the side of most prepackaged foods, below the major macronutrient list telling us the amount of carbohydrate, fat and protein, there will be a long list of ingredients made up of words we don't recognize that are difficult to pronounce.

Moreover, these are substances our bodies don't digest and assimilate well. If you take the time to research them, many are harmful and some are even cancer causing. Really? In my food and the food I feed my family, my children and grandchildren? Yes, it's all there and food manufacturers want you to know it (at least some of it). Why? Because of all these additives, they can provide you with what they call "wholesome goodness" that will survive on a store shelf for months and then on your pantry shelf for several more months. That should not make it OK. After all, the government is responsible for making sure that the food I can purchase is not harmful, is in fact healthful, and therefore I should have nothing to worry about. It really isn't as simple as all that.

For example, let's consider that many of these prepackaged foods contain wheat. Wheat, after all, is a mainstay. Wheat is mentioned several times in the Bible. The early Egyptians often had nothing more than bread and beer in their diets, both of which contained wheat. How can wheat be bad? After all, we've consumed it for centuries. This is all true. However, the wheat we eat today is far different from the wheat our ancestors ate. The wheat we eat now has been hybridized and altered to the point it doesn't even look the same.

If you stop and think for a minute, there may have been a time in your life, if you are old enough, when you would drive by wheat fields when the breeze was blowing. What a beautiful sight. You would see "amber waves of grain"; those golden-yellow stalks dancing in the breeze. We are hard-pressed to see such a wheat field these days. In fact, those wheat varieties some of us grew up with are now said to be of no economic value. They have adulterated wheat for various reasons. They now grow high-yield dwarf wheat, which was developed by cross-breeding and genetic manipulation around 1960. This adulteration of wheat has reduced those beautiful long, flowing stalks to ones measuring 18 to 24 inches. They are compacted and no longer able to dance in the breeze. Look at the kernels below and compare the size of those of ancient einkorn wheat with those of modern durum wheat. The einkorn wheat stalks are much longer and the kernels much smaller. This is the type of wheat that inspired "amber waves of grain." When was the last time you saw those beautiful fields of wheat? We don't see those now as hybridization has physically changed the appearance of wheat.

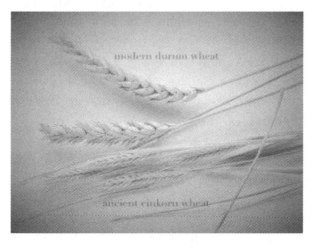

Figure 3 http://www.thehealthyhomeeconomist.com/wp-content/uploads/2012/06/einkornwheat2-300x241.jpg

In his book *Wheat Belly,* cardiologist and M.D. William Davis goes into significant detail about how wheat has been altered and its impact on our health, not only from a digestive perspective, but a cardiovascular perspective. He clearly outlines how wheat is processed in the body and how the glycemic index of whole grain wheat is more than that of white bread, a Mars bar, or even a Snickers bar. If you're someone who focuses on the glycemic index as an indicator of how certain foods elevate your blood sugar, it's very disheartening to learn that whole grain bread you spend good money on, to make that delicious sandwich, is not as good for you as you thought it was. It's even harmful. Dr. Davis discusses the effects of modern wheat and wheat gluten (the protein component of the wheat) on the vascular system, the impact wheat has on blood sugar levels (and consequently diabetes), as well as obesity, cardiovascular diseases like high blood pressure, kidney failure, and so on.[11]

William Davis is not the only one. In his book *Grain Brain,* neurologist and M.D. David Perlmutter paints an equally dismal picture of the ill effects of eating wheat, but from the neurological perspective. He talks about how wheat is a major contributor to many health concerns like ADD/ADHD, autism, Alzheimer's disease, dementia, and neuropathies, to name a few.[12] Both these men have observed the consequences of eating wheat as it relates to ill health and disease in their patients, and the dramatic improvements their patients see once wheat is removed from the diet.

In reading both of these books, two interesting facts stand out from my perspective. First, both of these physicians talk about how people can have significant medical conditions related to wheat without having digestive symptoms that would obviously indicate wheat is an issue. Secondly, neither of these men are gastroenterologists. One of the challenges I face working with clients each day is trying to get them to understand wheat can have a profoundly negative impact on health even if there isn't a digestive issue. They will tell me they don't have bloating, cramping, diarrhea, gas, etc. when they eat wheat and therefore assume without the physical digestive complaints, wheat does not bother them. In fact, that is just not true and the research is out there to show it.

What is it about wheat? Why is it so harmful? Why is it so different? How has it changed? The answers to these questions lie in the alterations and changes that have been made to wheat over the last 50 years or so. Genetic alterations and differences generated by thousands of human-engineered hybridizations has yielded significant variations in quality, composition, and appearance as shown in the picture above.

They tell us wheat has been hybridized and crossbred to be resistant to drought and parasites, and to provide increased yield per acre. During this hybridization the wheat gluten proteins undergo considerable structural changes. The end result is a gluten protein that is foreign to the human body. As wheat is the dominant source of gluten proteins in our diet, we have observed considerable problems in people as these proteins damage the gut lining, making it more permeable. This creates leaky gut syndrome and conditions like non-celiac gluten sensitivity and celiac disease. Celiac disease has been around a long time but, as noted earlier, there is a fourfold increase since the 1950s with fatal complications if not treated.

Also, consider that techniques used in the processing of wheat starting in the late 19th century made it possible to create massive amounts of refined wheat at a much lower cost. As a result the nutritious components of the grain, the bran and the germ, are separated from the endosperm, that portion where the starchy carbohydrates are contained, yielding a significant reduction in nutrient density. Further, this refined wheat causes rapid blood sugar spikes. Wheat just isn't what it used to be and it is not good for us from a beneficial nutrient standpoint.

So I'll stop eating bread, you say. Unfortunately that's just not enough. Gluten proteins are found not only in wheat but also in rye, barley, malt, spelt, and various other grains. There are higher amounts of gluten in some grains than others, which would make certain grains more tolerable. However, if you have gluten issues, you need to stay away from *all* gluten-containing grains. It becomes even more of a challenge to be gluten free.

Consider this: wheat and some of these other grains are used as fillers in most prepackaged foods. They are also in ice cream, soy sauce, prepared meats, soups and sauces, coffee substitutes, seitan (the fake meat vegans eat which is almost all gluten; that's what gives it a chewy consistency), candies like licorice, and other condiments. Now, would I tell a vegan to stop eating "vegan" meat? Of course not, but if that vegan has problems with gluten, a diet change might be in order.

So, after reading this you've made the decision to go gluten free. That doesn't seem so bad. You think to yourself, I can give up bread; I can give up those other things that have gluten in them. I can check my pet food to be sure it is gluten free. That way there is no chance of cross-contamination and my accidental exposure to anything with gluten in it. Maybe you find yourself thinking, there must be something to this. More and more people are talking about these problems and maybe there's more to this than you realized. There are certainly more and more "gluten-free" choices when I go to the grocery store. So I'll just look for those foods labeled "gluten-free."

Things are not always as they seem.

Genetically Modified Organisms

Now the real challenge begins. Many of those "gluten-free" foods sound healthy and are marketed to be a choice for you if gluten is an issue. They may even seem like a truly healthy choice. However, in many instances when these foods are made, there may be no wheat, but they instead contain genetically modified organisms (GMOs).

GMOs are living organisms whose genetic material has been altered. The genes have been manipulated in the laboratory through a process called genetic engineering. Crops are now engineered for insect resistance, fungal resistance, viral resistance, herbicide resistance, changed nutritional content, improved taste, and improved storage. This process is unlike cross breeding or hybridization, both of which involve related species. Genetic modification is the process of forcing genes from one species into another entirely unrelated species creating substances never before seen on earth.

One example is genetically modified (GM) corn, which is genetically engineered to produce its own insecticide that stays within the corn right up until the time you eat it. The corn used for food has been genetically modified to express the protein from *Bacillus thuringiensis* (Bt), that kills certain insects. The Bt is ingested by us when we eat corn. About 90 percent of the corn grown in the U.S. has been genetically modified, and about 90 percent of planted soybeans in the U.S. are genetically modified varieties.[13,14]

Some GM crops are genetically engineered to withstand being sprayed with Roundup®. These crops are referred to as "Roundup ready."

> **Example:** Corn + DNA from soil bacteria that is naturally immune to Roundup herbicide + E. coli bacteria + soil bacteria that causes tumors in plants (which enables the plant's cell wall to be breached) = Roundup Ready Corn (one of several Roundup Ready crops engineered by Monsanto).[15]

Roundup herbicide is sprayed on fields to kill weeds. It does so effectively because weeds contain the shikimate pathway, a metabolic pathway that is disrupted by the active ingredient in Roundup: *glyphosate*. Glyphosate is effective in killing off weeds, but the GM corn continues to grow because it has been genetically modified to withstand being sprayed. Further, the weeds are getting smart and are mutating requiring even more Roundup to be effective and achieve the desired "no weed" results.

The important thing to consider is all the time that crop is growing, it is pulling the glyphosate out of the soil into the plant. Therefore, when you eat GM corn, you eat glyphosate. Now Monsanto has always contended that glyphosate is not harmful to humans because human genes do not have the shikimate pathway.

In fact that is true, but recent research published in April 2013 in the journal *Entropy* demonstrates very clearly that each of the bacteria and microbes that live within our gut, and outnumber our own cells 10 to 1, *do* have the shikimate pathway. These same bacteria and microbes are responsible for sustaining us, as will be discussed in great detail later in this book. Glyphosate disrupts the gut bacteria's pathway, the same way it does the plant's pathway. In fact, it is more disruptive to the gut's population of beneficial bacteria than the gut's population of pathogens, or less desirable microbes as I refer to them. This allows gut pathogens to overgrow creating excess toxins.[16]

The production of these excess toxins leads to systemic inflammation, and inflammation of the gut itself, which leads to leaky gut syndrome. The report goes on to specifically cite the link between the effects of glyphosate on the gut bacteria and the subsequent relationship to those frequently reported conditions like autism, neurological problems, Alzheimer's disease, allergies, cardiovascular problems, autoimmune diseases, diabetes, obesity, infertility, and so on.

So if you read your labels and find things like soy protein isolate, textured soy protein, soy flour, soy lecithin, corn solids, corn syrup, high fructose corn syrup, or maltodextrin, chances are you're eating genetically modified foods. Maltodextrin is frequently seen. Maltodextrin is a filler and although there are other sources, that do not come from GM corn, like potato, rice or tapioca, most maltodextrin in prepackaged food is from GM corn. Unless the product says "USDA Organic," the soy or the corn or any part thereof, is most likely GM. If GM corn or soy are used in a product, that product cannot display the label "USDA Organic."

Some food manufacturers recognize the potential concerns people have regarding GM foods and the importance of keeping consumers informed. If there are no GMOs in their prepackaged food items, they will be labeled "Non-GMO." This is not something they must do. In fact there has been a big push over the last several years to force food manufacturers to label foods that contain GMOs. The feeling on the part of educated consumers is they have a right to know if they are eating foods they feel may be potentially harmful.

However, companies like Monsanto, the major player with respect to the research and development of GMOs, and other chemical companies who stand to gain from the sale of all the chemicals sprayed on our foods, do not want consumers to know. They fear if they are told there are GMOs in the food, they probably won't buy the foods. If they don't know for sure, they don't have the time to sort it all out, so the food will probably sell. Those who are aware may choose not to purchase or consume those foods but who really has the time to check it all out.

Researchers blame GMOs and glyphosate for many health challenges as noted above. I find the research to be very revealing and believable. We have seen the numbers of people with at least three chronic diseases increase dramatically over the last several years. There must be a reason; or several reasons and they seem to be linked to our foods.

There are two sides to this story, and some are content to believe the government has our best interest in mind and would not let food manufacturers produce and market products that might be harmful to U.S. consumers. Clearly, the Food and Drug Administration (FDA) would have us believe they are protecting us. Part of their mission statement tells us:

> FDA is responsible for protecting the public health by assuring the safety, efficacy and security of human and veterinary drugs, biological products, medical devices, our nation's food supply, cosmetics, and products that emit radiation.[17]

Some feel that is just not true.

Research on the part of consumer advocacy groups, as well as many concerned parents and grandparents who investigate and study information because of their concerns, calls into question the steps being taken by those who claim to have our best interest at heart. When data such as that recorded on the graph below become common knowledge, educated and concerned citizens start to question who the FDA is really looking out for.

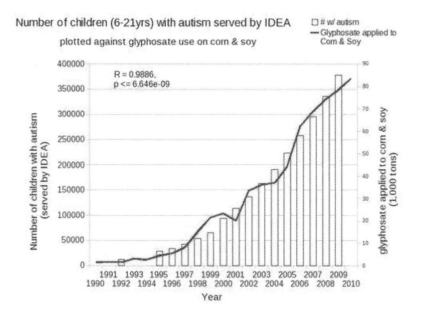

Number of children (6-21yrs) with autism served by IDEA
plotted against glyphosate use on corn & soy

□ # w/ autism
— Glyphosate applied to Corn & Soy

Figure 4 http://www.examiner.com/article/data-show-correlations-between-increase-neurological-diseases-and-gmos

In his newly released book *Altered Genes, Twisted Truth*, Steven M. Drucker helps set the record straight.[18] He goes into great detail providing an accurate historical record of the irresponsible behavior of many eminent scientists and scientific institutions in the earlier decades of the genetic engineering revolution. I have studied GMO and the information about the inherent dangers and I am aware of the revolving door between the FDA and Monsanto.

However, this book opened my eyes to information known from long before the days of

Michael Taylor and the others I am aware of involved in trying to convince us it is all good, and in our best interest. According to Drucker:

> Contrary to the assertions of its proponents, the massive enterprise to reconfigure the genetic core of the world's food supply is not based on sound science but on the systematic subversion of science—and it would collapse if subjected to an open airing of the facts.

As a person who looks at these facts, I am concerned.

Now to confuse the issue just a little more, many food manufacturers will label a product organic. If you purchase foods with the USDA's official organic seal, you should be able to assume several things are true about that food. It will have been grown without synthetic fertilizers and pesticides, sewage sludge, or irradiation, and it won't contain genetically modified organisms. Meat labeled organic will have been raised on crops held to the same standard and will be free of antibiotics, steroids, and growth hormones. The animal will have been handled according to certain standards on animal health and welfare pre-slaughter, and not stressed right up until the moment of slaughter. You should expect the same high quality of foods other than produce and meat that bear the same label. But what about those foods labeled simply "Organic"? There are many of them out there.

Herein lies the fallacy. "Organic" does not necessarily mean 100 percent organic, or that it's healthy and good for you. In his recently released book *Organic: A Journalist's Quest to Discover the Truth behind Food Labeling*, Peter Laufer, Ph.D. chronicles his quest to find the truth about some walnuts and some beans labeled "Organic."[19] The story is well-written and uncovers much about what the food industry really does to convince us they are marketing only the best to us as consumers. Some of the facts he uncovered were very disappointing, to say the least. Will I go so far as to say "You can't trust anyone"? No, but I do encourage you to walk away with the knowledge that all is not as it seems, especially when you are buying "Organic." Perhaps some aspect of that "healthy" food is organic, but the remaining ingredients may not be organic.

Further, we are learning some foods labeled "organic" and "Non-GMO" are not. My family and I really enjoy corn chips with salsa made from my own freshly grown veggies and herbs (living in Texas for 20 years, I learned to make it the right way). We stopped eating that delicious salsa with corn chips many years ago because, after all, they were corn and at the time 88 percent of the corn in this country was reported to be GM.

Fast forward to a few years ago when a friend who knew of my love of chips and salsa shared with me the great new corn chips she had discovered. They were in a nondescript brown bag that claimed, right on the front, in red letters, "No Gluten" and "No GMO." Could it really be? Could I once again enjoy my all-time favorite snack? The answer to the less well-informed self was a resounding, YES. How could these be anything but good? After all there it was, right on the front of the bag. We again began to enjoy chips and salsa every chance we could, and I would always go out of my way to ensure my friends and extended family I was watching out for them; I had their best interest in mind. "These chips are healthy; just read the label. It says right here, in red letters." My favorite snack was healthy again.

Imagine my dismay when I learned these facts a few months ago. Not only were these chips not non-GMO, the *Consumer Reports* investigation found they contained over 75 percent GMO corn, after testing 6 different bags.[20] It was reported both the supplier and the manufacturer were surprised by the results. At least the white variety met non-GMO standards. The conclusion from this study was that purchasing products with the Non-GMO Project Verified seal was best as all products tested and marketed with that seal, met non-GMO standards.

Learning to Read Food Labels

It has become common practice for many to pick up a prepackaged food and read the label. Some are looking for how many carbs or how much fat, but the one often misinterpreted section is, calories per serving and serving size. Below are two nutrition facts panels. The one on the left has been used for the last 20 years and next to it is the proposed new panel. Looking at the currently used panel, the word "calories" is in bold letters but the actual number is not. Looking at the proposed panel, both "calories" and the number are bold, and the number is larger. Often consumers look at the calories and see only 230. Unless they understand that is 230 calories per serving, and that a serving is only 2/3 of a cup, they might think the 230 is for the entire container and never think twice about eating the entire thing. In this case, that might be extreme as there are 8 servings per container, but you get the idea.

Nutrition Facts	
Serving Size 2/3 cup (55g)	
Servings Per Container About 8	
Amount Per Serving	
Calories 230	Calories from Fat 72
	% Daily Value*
Total Fat 8g	**12%**
Saturated Fat 1g	**5%**
Trans Fat 0g	
Cholesterol 0mg	**0%**
Sodium 160mg	**7%**
Total Carbohydrate 37g	**12%**
Dietary Fiber 4g	**16%**
Sugars 1g	
Protein 3g	
Vitamin A	10%
Vitamin C	8%
Calcium	20%
Iron	45%

* Percent Daily Values are based on a 2,000 calorie diet. Your daily value may be higher or lower depending on your calorie needs.

	Calories:	2,000	2,500
Total Fat	Less than	65g	80g
Sat Fat	Less than	20g	25g
Cholesterol	Less than	300mg	300mg
Sodium	Less than	2,400mg	2,400mg
Total Carbohydrate		300g	375g
Dietary Fiber		25g	30g

Nutrition Facts	
8 servings per container	
Serving size	2/3 cup (55g)
Amount per 2/3 cup	
Calories	**230**
	% DV*
12%	**Total Fat** 8g
5%	Saturated Fat 1g
	Trans Fat 0g
0%	**Cholesterol** 0mg
7%	**Sodium** 160mg
12%	**Total Carbs** 37g
14%	Dietary Fiber 4g
	Sugars 1g
	Added Sugars 0g
	Protein 3g
10%	Vitamin D 2mcg
20%	Calcium 260mg
45%	Iron 8mg
5%	Potassium 235mg

* Footnote on Daily Values (DV) and calories reference to be inserted here.

Figure 3 http://www.fda.gov/Food/GuidanceRegulation/GuidanceDocuments Regulatory Information/LabelingNutrition/ucm385663.htm#images

Let's consider some other examples. Below is the panel off a canister of mixed nuts. I like nuts. I consider them a good source of some healthy fats and proteins.

When I eat nuts I have to be careful, as many people do, because a handful is good, a second handful better, and so on until they are all gone. But there are 190 calories in ¼ cup if I read the panel, and ¼ cup really isn't much.

Nutrition Facts

Serving Size 1oz.(28g)
Servings Per Container 10

Amount Per Serving
Calories: 190 Calories from fat: 160

	% Daily Value*
Total Fat: 17 g	26%
Saturated Fat 3 g	15%
Trans Fat 0 g	
Cholesterol: 0 mg	0%
Sodium: 135 mg	6%
Total Carbohydrates: 7 g	2%
Dietary Fiber: 2 g	8%
Sugars: 2 g	
Protein: 5 g	

Vitamin A: 0%	Vitamin C: 1%
Calciuim: 3%	Iron: 6%

*Percent Daily Values are based on a 2,000 calorie diet.

10 oz. Mixed Nuts

Let's consider the next example. This is the nutrition facts panel from a box of a popular toaster pastry. Now, I would never suggest someone eat these toaster pastries. They have that long list of ingredients in print so small you can't read it, and despite the fact the big yellow bubble found on the front of some of the boxes draws your attention to the fact these delightful treats are a "Good Source of 7 Vitamins and Minerals," in my world, they are not food; not really.

As a matter of example, though, think about this. Have you ever eaten the popular toaster pastry or perhaps given your children or grandchildren that toaster pastry warm from the toaster? I would venture to guess you did not open the foil pouch, remove one pastry, and neatly fold over the ends to close the pouch and save the second pastry for another day. Not likely and probably not something you would ever consider doing. No, they taste so good, you'll just eat both.

While you are trying to get through the grocery store, or perhaps during that endless moment while your impatient child is waiting for the toaster to pop, you glance at the nutrition panel on the side of the box and see 200 calories. That's not so bad, you tell yourself. All the energy he or she has will work off those 200 calories.

Look more closely. That 200 calories is the amount *per serving* and the "serving size" is 1 pastry. What a surprise this is for many people. This is the way nutrition facts panels work. The information is there regarding calories and serving size, but you need to know what you're looking for. This is a small part of the reason why we have become increasingly obese and unhealthy as a nation.

Nutrition Facts

Serving Size   1 Pastry (50g)

Amount Per Serving

Calories 200   Calories from Fat 45

	% Daily Value*
Total Fat 5g	**8%**
Saturated Fat 2g	**10%**
Trans Fat 0g	
Polyunsaturated Fat 1g	
Monounsaturated Fat 2g	
Cholesterol 0mg	**0%**
Sodium 240mg	**10%**
Total Carbohydrate 36g	**12%**
Dietary Fiber less than 1g	**4%**
Sugars 19g	
Protein 2g	

Vitamin A   10% • Vitamin C   0% • Calcium   0% • Iron   10%

Thiamin   10% • Riboflavin 10% • Niacin   10% • Vitamin B6 10%

* Percent Daily Values are based on a 2,000 calorie diet. Your daily values may be higher or lower depending on your calorie needs:

	Calories	2,000	2,500
Total Fat	Less than	65g	80g
Sat. Fat	Less than	20g	25g
Cholesterol	Less than	300mg	300mg
Sodium	Less than	2,400mg	2,400mg
Total Carbohydrate		300g	375g
Dietary Fiber		25g	30g

Calories per gram: Fat   9   •   Carbohydrate   4   •   Protein   4

INGREDIENTS: ENRICHED FLOUR (WHEAT FLOUR, NIACIN, REDUCED IRON, VITAMIN B1 [THIAMIN MONONITRATE], VITAMIN B2 [RIBOFLAVIN], FOLIC ACID), CORN SYRUP, SUGAR, HIGH FRUCTOSE CORN SYRUP, PALM OIL (WITH TBHQ FOR FRESHNESS), PEANUT BUTTER (PEANUTS, PEANUT OIL, TBHQ FOR FRESHNESS), SEMISWEET CHOCOLATE (SUGAR, CHOCOLATE, DEXTROSE), GLYCERIN, CONTAINS TWO PERCENT OR LESS OF FRUCTOSE, MODIFIED CORN STARCH, SALT, COCOA (PROCESSED WITH ALKALI), LEAVENING (BAKING SODA, SODIUM ACID PYROPHOSPHATE, MONOCALCIUM PHOSPHATE), CARAMEL COLOR, NATURAL AND ARTIFICIAL FLAVOR, SOY PROTEIN, GELATIN, POTASSIUM SORBATE (PRESERVATIVE), MONO- AND DIGLYCERIDES, DEXTROSE, SODIUM STEAROYL LACTYLATE, DATEM, COLOR ADDED, SOY LECITHIN, YELLOW 5 LAKE, CARRAGEENAN, RED 40 LAKE, VITAMIN A PALMITATE, NIACINAMIDE, BLUE 1 LAKE, REDUCED IRON, RED 40, VITAMIN B6 (PYRIDOXINE HYDROCHLORIDE), NONFAT MILK, ALMOND BUTTER (ALMONDS), VITAMIN B2 (RIBOFLAVIN), VITAMIN B1 (THIAMIN HYDROCHLORIDE).

**CONTAINS WHEAT, PEANUT, MILK, SOY
AND ALMOND INGREDIENTS.**

CHAPTER 3

YOU ARE WHAT YOU DIGEST

When I was growing up we used to say, "You are what you eat." I can remember teasing that if you ate a piece of chocolate cake it would show up on your hips. Today, it is more correct to say you are what you digest, or absorb or assimilate. That is because so much of what we consume when eating the Standard American Diet, or SAD diet (as many call it), cannot be broken down and assimilated by the human body. Those unidentifiable ingredients on the nutrition facts panel are often not fit for human consumption. The body simply cannot break them down and does not know what to do with them.

You might ask, "Is the body really that smart?" I will say yes, and also tell you the body struggles trying to get the nutrients it needs from many of the foods you might eat.

Think about it like this. You are reading this at the present time, at your present stage in life. No matter who you are, you are not the same in physical form that you were when you were born, or when you were two years old, and so on. You have changed. You may have the same DNA, but physically you have grown taller, broader, most likely smarter, and certainly more aware. This did not happen without eating food and having those foods broken down into the molecular structures necessary to build you to become who you are. Bone, muscles, teeth, hair, fingernails, organs, and tissues have all grown as a result of your body doing what it needed to do with the food it was given. If you have maintained healthy eating habits all of your life, chances are very good you are physically healthy. Your hair shines, you have healthy looking skin, your eyes are bright, you don't have problems with your weight, and you have a healthy relationship with others in your world.

If, on the other hand, you have not eaten such a healthy diet and have perhaps attempted to sustain yourself on the SAD diet, you may, in fact, not be so healthy. You may have noticed things like your hair doesn't shine, so you buy many different expensive hair care products to make it shine. Maybe your skin isn't healthy, so you spend much of your hard-earned money to treat or cover up the blemishes and the blotches and the age spots. After all, don't those commercials—the ones with exquisitely beautiful models showing shiny hair and airbrushed skin—say their products will work?

What about your weight? Have you tried every diet out there only to find that none of them really work? Let's face it, if weight reduction programs worked, there would not be a new one on the market every other week and there certainly would not be millions of dollars to be made by people promoting their programs. Some work for some, but most only work with a lot of commitment on the part of the dieter. And those that do work, usually are designed around healthy, whole food and not much of what you find in the SAD diet.

Then there's the relationship part. This is a very important part of life for everyone. If you are chronically tired, cranky, irritable, frustrated, rushed, short-tempered, unable to sleep well at night, unable to awaken refreshed in the morning full of energy and ready to face the day with a smile on your face and a bounce in your step, it is probably because of what you eat and drink (or what you don't eat and drink).

Hippocrates, often referred to as the "father of medicine" said, "Let food be thy medicine and medicine be thy food." That was some 2000 years ago. He wasn't talking about the food most of us eat today and I suspect he would never have imagined what modern man has done to food.

How Does Digestion Work?

Let's start at the beginning.

The entire process of eating and digesting food so it will be available for energy—to help us move, think, and function in a healthful way—is complicated by the fact eating has become too easy.

Now, there are some who might argue with that statement and they are the ones who would say, "Who has time to fix dinner?" Giving this some thought, do you eat to live or live to eat? Is what you are looking at to eat at any given moment something that will nourish your body? Is it instead something that will satisfy a craving (because you are nutritionally deficient) or satisfy a desire because you haven't tasted something like that for quite a while?

Consider that during the days of the hunter-gatherer, food was as important as breathing or sleeping to keep a person healthy. Many hours each day were spent to ensure there was life-sustaining food available for self and family. Today, the act of hunting and gathering is a trip to the grocery store where things are neatly laid out for us and we pick and choose what looks good. Or, in our rush, we drive to the local fast-food window and order what we want from, often an extensive menu of prepared foods, and go on about our day. This activity is harmful in more ways than just consuming fast food.

Interestingly, the first phase of digestion is the *cephalic* phase. Cephalic relates to the head and, in this case, the brain. This phase, also called *vagus nerve stimulation*, is the first of three phases of digestion and happens even before we start eating. The vagus nerve is the longest of the cranial nerves, originating in the brain and extending from the brain to the abdomen. During this phase, the brain begins to prepare the body for digestion. The vagus nerve sends signals to the brain indicating it is time to prepare for digestion. During this phase the sight, the smell, the taste or simply the thought of food will make your mouth water.

Take a minute, right now, close your eyes, and think of your favorite food. It doesn't matter what it is; just visualize your favorite food. In the brief few seconds it took for you to do that, chances are your mouth began to water. During the cephalic phase of digestion as the brain begins to stimulate the body to prepare to break down, digest, and absorb nutrients, many things are happening. Signals are stimulating and initiating the flow of gastric secretions, specifically pepsin and hydrochloric acid so the stomach is ready when the food arrives.

During this phase the pancreas is also stimulated to start producing the enzymes necessary to assist in the breaking down of food molecules into smaller molecules, which can then be taken by way of the bloodstream to go and do the jobs that need to be done throughout the rest of the body. These actions are all necessary to ensure the food we take in is adequately broken down and properly utilized.

This cephalic phase is a very important phase of digestion and one that we often don't experience adequately because we are often eating on the run. Before the advent of convenience foods and drive-through lanes, meals were prepared and often baked in the oven. All the time they were baking, the smells that filled the home and made our mouth water, were actually doing so much more. Your body does not have the opportunity to experience the benefits of this phase of digestion if you are zipping through a fast food restaurant line or zapping something in the microwave oven (something I don't recommend). Either way, our bodies don't have the proper digestive experience. This actually sets up a situation where the food arrives in the stomach, but the stomach is not ready for the task at hand. Remember, all of this activity should be happening *before* we start eating.

The Mouth—It's Not Just for Talking

When we eat, we put food into our mouths and the chewing process begins. Tasting the food will stimulate the cephalic phase as noted above, but let's take a minute to talk about the physical act of chewing.

You have probably been told sometime along the way, you should chew your food 30 times before you swallow it. Now there are several good reasons for this and I am sure if you are reading this and you are not in the habit of chewing 30 times you may question what I am saying. Most people don't chew 30 times and that is because they are either eating too quickly, or there is not enough substance to do so. If your diet is the Standard American Diet (SAD) diet, and the foods you are eating are pre-processed and pre-packaged, they are loaded with fillers, starches, and carbohydrates, mostly from GMO corn. A certain enzyme made by the salivary glands in your mouth, *salivary amylase*, will immediately start acting on those starches and carbohydrates. That's what enzymes do. They break down the food they are specifically created to act on. In the case of the foods eaten in the SAD diet, there is very little real whole food, it is loaded with fillers, and you would be hard pressed to chew 30 times.

Chewing is very important and if the foods you're eating are whole foods, in addition to adding the salivary amylase, the process will break the large pieces of food into much smaller particles increasing the surface area of the food. These smaller particles will then be acted on more efficiently by the gastric juices once they hit the stomach. The act of chewing also forms the food into a *bolus* and lubricates it for the trip down the esophagus and into the stomach.

Taking the time to chew 30 times may also allow you to feel satiated more quickly and may in fact contribute to your eating less. *Ghrelin* is a hormone produced in the stomach and in the pancreas. Among other things, ghrelin hormone production stimulates hunger. As we eat, Ghrelin production slows, we feel less hungry and if we have been eating more slowly, will feel satiated more quickly.[21]

Swallowing—Getting Food and Drink from the Mouth to the Stomach

I mention swallowing as it is also important and there are key things to keep in mind as food gets from the mouth to the stomach. The process of swallowing is a complex neuromuscular activity that allows for the safe transport of material from the mouth to the stomach for digestion without compromising the airway.[22]

During swallowing, the goal is to move food into the esophagus, keeping it out of the respiratory system. Picking the correct tunnel, if you will. Several events occur rapidly and often simultaneously during this process. Food is propelled from the front to the back of the mouth as the lips and sides of the tongue direct it efficiently toward the *pharynx* (the tunnel that connects the mouth with the esophagus). Over 20 muscles in the mouth, throat, and esophagus are involved and are governed in part by swallowing centers in the brain stem. For the most part, it is not something we consciously think about when eating, unless we choke, or unless the person trying to swallow has had some type of brain injury or stroke. In the hospital I've cared for many stroke patients who must be told to swallow. This happens when the normal swallow mechanism no longer works if that part of the brain is affected by the stroke.

Muscles in the pharynx contract in a peristaltic wave and this moves the bolus downward. The soft palate, the back of the roof of the mouth raises to prevent the bolus of food from refluxing into the nasal cavity. If you've ever choked while eating or drinking and had fluid come up through your nose, it was because the soft palate was unable to do its job while you were choking. Muscles and structures in this area function to ensure the epiglottis (the cartilaginous structure that keeps food from going into the wrong tunnel), protects the airway so the food moves down and not back up; into the esophagus and not into the lungs. Peristaltic movement of the esophagus, which is a muscular tube, carries the bolus of food downward into the stomach. Once the food reaches the stomach, the lower esophageal sphincter closes to prevent gastro esophageal reflux, or the backing up of food into the esophagus.

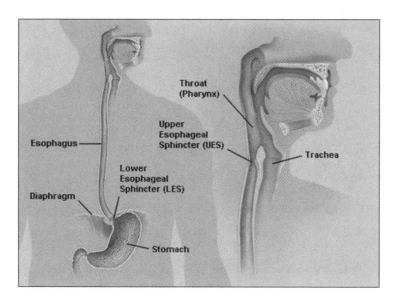

Figure 5 http://1.yukozimo.com/no/3136-1.jpg

If you are eating slowly and chewing properly, you should be able to swallow each mouthful of well-chewed food without the aid of a drink.

The Esophagus—Not So Interesting in My Opinion, But Warrants Discussion

I talk about the esophagus as my least favorite part of the digestive system. In my mind, it is simply a conduit from the mouth to the stomach. There is the peristalsis that keeps food moving downward, as well as the mucus that's produced to facilitate that movement, but there are no active enzymes produced in the esophagus. The only enzyme activity going on in the esophagus is because of the enzymes in the whole foods eaten, the enzymes added to food while it was in the mouth, or the digestive enzymes taken before meals as a supplement.

At the end of the esophagus is a ring-shaped muscle called the lower esophageal sphincter (LES), also called the cardiac sphincter, which, along with the diaphragmatic sphincter works as a valve to keep things in the stomach. Conventional medicine has studied these and surrounding structures to answer function questions and to help develop new surgical techniques to be considered when these sphincters are not working properly.

From my perspective, they are sphincters and therefore, they are muscles and if they are not working properly, it may have more to so with a nutritional deficiency, namely the minerals calcium and magnesium, than an anatomical mishap that needs to be corrected.

I am not discounting the actual fact a poorly functioning lower esophageal sphincter (LES) can be problematic. Millions of people take the "little purple pill" or another type of antacid medication every day to help with the problems and symptoms they suffer because these sphincter muscles are not working properly.

Medications given if a person has a problem or symptoms like acid indigestion or gastro esophageal reflux disease (GERD) are not designed to correct the problem with sphincter control. These drugs act to either neutralize the acid or limit acid production so when the sphincter doesn't clamp closed, and gastric contents containing hydrochloric acid (HCl) reflux into the esophagus, that acid will not injure the esophageal lining. If GERD is a problem, conventional medicine recommends lifestyle changes.

These include don't eat foods that cause the problem, don't drink alcohol, don't overeat, don't lie down after eating, and take a drug. If a lesser drug fails a stronger drug will be substituted. When that drug fails, there's always the consideration for surgery. The surgeries are relatively uncomplicated. During the procedure the upper part of the stomach is actually wrapped around the esophagus and sewn in place so the esophagus now passed through a tube of stomach muscle. This is to keep acid from regurgitating up into the esophagus as easily.

Because I have experienced great results myself taking healthy supplements, I compare these procedures to removing the engine because the car is not running, when all that was really needed was gas in the tank.

All of these approaches are not without potential complications. Certainly a surgical procedure comes with risks, though relatively uncomplicated. Taking these medications will also cause problems. Conventional medicine prescribes the drug and recommends the lifestyle changes. These drugs are to be used short-term while the lifestyle changes help to correct the problem.

Antacid medications were first prescribed starting back in the 1970s. As time has gone on, we have learned that there are significant complications associated with long-term use of these drugs. Research has revealed concerns associated with antacid use to include impaired nutrient absorption especially protein absorption, deficiencies of critical nutrients such as B12, calcium, iron, magnesium, and so on. In addition, without HCl you lose the first line of defense against food-borne bacteria.

This increases the risk of bacterial overgrowth in the stomach and, ultimately, the intestines, not to mention an increased risk of infection, cancer, and other diseases. Yet, some people take these drugs for years (despite the fact the package insert clearly states for short term use and lists all the potential complications) refilling the prescription each month, because without the drugs, the symptoms will return. "But my doctor says..."

Wow, maybe taking those drugs isn't such a good idea. Consider this. Soft drink consumption disrupts the normal acid-base balance in your stomach. That's right, if you drink soft drinks, you're interfering with normal acid production, stomach function and digestion. The phosphoric acid in soft drinks interacts with stomach acid, slowing digestion and blocking nutrient absorption. It interferes with the body's ability to absorb calcium and can lead to osteoporosis, cavities and bone softening. Sounds like a recipe for osteoarthritis and possibly joint replacement surgery.

Let's go to a nice restaurant and order a blue cheeseburger. While waiting for the meal, consume a carbonated beverage. Several things will happen: the carbonation will start to make your stomach bloat and, as noted above, the phosphoric acid will interact with the stomach acid. By the time your burger arrives, you might as well throw it in the trash for all the nutritional benefit you'll get.

Because of the healthy acid disruption, you will not be able to break down the initial bonds of protein in the meat or cheese, you will not be able to assimilate the B vitamins from the lettuce, you will not be able to assimilate the calcium from the cheese, or iron, magnesium and other trace minerals and nutrients that might otherwise be available in that burger with the blue cheese. We won't take the time to talk about what eating the bread or using the condiments will do right now.

What can you do if you suffer with GERD? The pain and the symptoms are terrible, I know. I suffered from a mild case for several years. For me it would act up especially if I had eaten chocolate, had coffee, or if I was overtired. I had a particularly tough time while I was pregnant.

Fortunately for me, while sharing my concerns with a naturopathic friend, I was reminded of the importance of the lower esophageal sphincter as a muscle. As a muscle, it must contract and close tightly to keep the gastric contents down in the stomach. Like all muscles in the body, this muscle requires calcium and magnesium to function properly. My approach was to increase my good quality calcium/magnesium intake and add some digestive enzymes, taken with my meals. GERD has not been a problem for me for several years.

The Stomach—The Churning Factory: Mixing It All Together

The stomach is often described as a J-shaped tube, sometimes a crescent, and sometimes simply as an enlargement of the gastrointestinal tract. When the stomach is empty, it is about the size of a large sausage. Anatomically, it is located at the end of the esophagus and is in the left upper portion of the abdomen. It is connected to the esophagus on the upper end and the duodenum, or first part of the small intestine, on the lower end. I mentioned the cephalic phase of digestion which is the first phase of gastric juice production. The second phase of gastric juice production begins in the stomach.

Food enters the stomach, causing it to stretch. This in turn sends nervous impulses to the brain. The brain then sends return impulses back to the stomach to begin secreting *gastrin*. Gastrin is a hormone that stimulates the release of other gastric juices. The stomach continually secretes these gastric juices and is responsible for the production of approximately two to three quarts (liters) of gastric juices every day. Therefore, the specific functions of the stomach are the temporary storage and mixing of food, the secretion of gastric juices into the *lumen* (the body of the stomach) and the release of the hormone gastrin into the blood.

The wall of the stomach consists of four layers. The outer layer is called the peritoneal layer. It is part of the *peritoneum*, the membrane that lines the inside of the abdomen, covering most of the organs. This layer does not play a role in digestion. There is also a muscular layer, made up of a longitudinal layer, a circular layer, and an oblique layer of muscle fibers. The *submucosa* layer is a mucous layer of membrane that forms the inner lining. The muscles in the muscular coat account for the fact the stomach is able to expand when food enters it. The muscle fibers slide over one another, reducing the thickness of the stomach wall while actually increasing the stomach area. So the stomach expands while the active breakdown of food is going on and contracts when no food is present. The contraction of these muscles when the stomach is empty stimulates nerves in the wall of the stomach that contribute to the sensation of hunger pangs.

The muscles of the stomach contract in rhythm when food enters the stomach. This combined action sends a series of wavelike contractions from the upper portion of the stomach to the lower end. These gentle, rippling waves or contractions pass over the stomach every 15 to 25 seconds and are known as *peristalsis*. This peristaltic action begins to mix the partially digested food with the stomach secretions and any ingested liquid until it has the consistency of a thick soup. This thick soup material is known as *chyme*. The contractions continue to push this mixture a few milliliters at a time into the small intestine.

The part of the stomach where the contents empty out of the esophagus is called the *cardia*. Above and to the left of the opening of the stomach is the portion called the *fundus*. When food enters the stomach, it resides in the fundus or upper portion as the body of the stomach prepares itself for digestion. The fundus contains cells that produce the acid, and pepsin, the chief digestive enzyme in the stomach responsible for breaking down proteins. Food gets mixed and held in the fundus where enzymatic digestion starts, provided there are live active enzymes in the food you've eaten, or you take a digestive enzyme supplement before your meal. Stomach acid is released into the fundus, but at about 30 percent concentration so it will not affect enzymatic digestion. The food remains in the fundus for about 40 to 60 minutes. Up to 75 percent of digestion can take place during this phase, provided there are enough enzymes available.

I will talk much more about enzymes later, but for now, realize that if you're eating raw, organic fruits and vegetables, or even better if you are juicing these fruits and vegetables, you are giving your body the benefit of live active enzymes available in that food. If all the food you're eating has been cooked, there are no live active enzymes in that food because taking food to a temperature above 118°F will kill all live active enzymes.

The fundus is one primary site of ghrelin production, the hormone that stimulates hunger. As food entering the fundus stretches the stomach, ghrelin production slows. Ghrelin levels increase prior to meals and are suppressed postprandially (following a meal) in proportion to the amount of calories ingested.[23]

When this cycle is complete, the thick soup type material known as *chyme* moves down into the body of the stomach. If there were plenty of enzymes available while in the fundus, the molecules of food are adequately broken down. In the body of the stomach HCl is released at full levels. Once in the body of the stomach, churning and mixing begins in earnest.

Only a small amount of mixing goes on in the fundus, that's primarily the site of enzymatic breakdown if the enzymes are available. This helps us understand the importance of enzymes because if the food has not been acted on appropriately by enzymes in the fundus, it enters the body of the stomach inefficiently broken down. The muscles are working vigorously to mix up the food and it continues to churn and roll over and over within the stomach as this mixing continues.

Once the mixing is complete, the food then enters the portion of the stomach called the *antrum* where it is held up briefly. Food then leaves the antrum of the stomach entering the first part of the small intestine, the *duodenum,* through the pyloric sphincter at the end of the stomach. The food is not dumped into the duodenum all at once; it actually leaves a few milliliters at a time. The pyloric sphincter muscle relaxes to allow the flow of chyme out of the antrum of the stomach, then contracts, initiating a backward pressure into the stomach which continues to mix up the contents. The stomach itself empties in approximately 1 to 4 hours depending upon the foods that have been eaten. Foods rich in carbohydrates leave the stomach more rapidly than proteins and proteins leave more rapidly than fats.

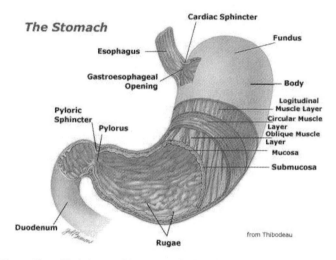

Figure 6 http://devindevon.wikispaces.com/file/view/stomach2.jpg/301997910/ 392x297/stomach2.jpg

There is also a major chemical digestion that takes place within the stomach. The *mucosa* is a layer of epithelial cells forming columns of secretory cells called gastric glands within the stomach lining. Secretions flow into the stomach from these glands. Gastric glands actually contain three types of exocrine gland cells that secrete juices into the stomach lumen. These are mucous neck cells, the parietal cells and the chief cells as shown below. Both surface mucous cells and mucous neck cells are responsible for secreting mucus. It is this mucus that provides the protection of the lining of the stomach from its harsh acidic environment.

Remember, the acid in the stomach is HCl, the same acid that put holes in your jeans in the chemistry lab. Without the protection of the mucus on the inside lining of the stomach, the acid would eat a hole through the stomach wall.

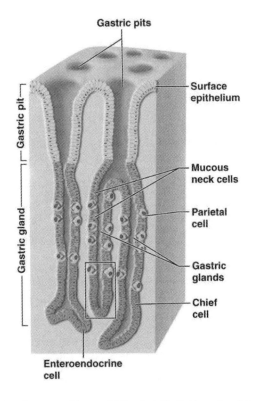

Figure 7 http://www.angelfire.com/ok3/apologia/drafts/stomach_cell.jpg

Stomach acid is created by *parietal* cells. These cells secrete hydrogen ions and chloride ions both into the stomach lumen. When the time is right these ions come together and produce the HCl. The strong acidic fluid kills many microbes in food (making it the first line of defense against foodborne bacteria) and partially breaks down the proteins in food. HCl also provides the best environment for the pepsin (an enzyme synthesized in its inactive form in the stomach) to work. HCl denatures the protein and begins to unfold protein molecules so the pepsin can do its job most efficiently. Without adequate amounts of HCl, that initial breakdown of protein does not happen efficiently.

HCl also stimulates the secretion of hormones that promote the flow of bile and pancreatic juices. Gastrin is a hormone produced by the G cells in the lining of the stomach and upper portion of the small intestine. Before we eat, in anticipation of a meal, nerves in the brain are stimulated and they signal the stomach to begin to release gastrin. The gastrin is also released when the stomach is stretched. So, gastrin stimulates the production *cholecystokinin* (CCK) responsible for promoting the flow of bile and pancreatic juices and the major hormone that regulates acid secretion in the stomach.

The chief cells are responsible for the secretion of *pepsinogen,* the inactive precursor of pepsin, and gastric lipase. Pepsin as noted above is the enzyme responsible for the initial breakdown of protein molecules into smaller peptides initiating enzymatic digestion of proteins in the stomach. The only proteolytic (protein digesting) enzyme found in the stomach is pepsin which is secreted by the chief cells. Pepsin is only effective in a very acidic environment in the stomach, a good reason why ample amounts of stomach acid must be present. This is the only way the pepsin does its job and ensures the initial breakdown of protein. Otherwise, the inadequate initial breakdown of proteins will cause significant problems later on, as we will see.

Let's Talk Enzymes—
The Foundation of Life

First, we recognize that there are different types of enzymes and enzyme systems in the body. We have digestive, metabolic, and food enzymes and they are the most important elements of life. Without enzymes available to "make it happen," *nothing* in the human body will function. While you read this book your heart beats, you breathe in and out, your hair is growing, your fingernails are growing, and if you've eaten recently, the meal is being digested, and so on. Each of these jobs within the human body requires a massive amount of enzymatic activity to make the job happen.

So what are enzymes? Enzymes are biological catalysts responsible for supporting almost all of the biochemical reactions that maintain homeostasis in the body. They are:

- Proteins that hold an electrical charge
- Catalysts, substances that speed up the reaction but do not get used up in the process

- Specific in that they only cleave or cut certain bonds
- In the case of digestive enzymes, efficient in that one enzyme can break down millions of bonds

Digestive enzymes are specific for the various components of food they are designed to break down. The major types of digestive enzymes are:

- Amylase—will break down carbohydrates, starches, and sugars which are prevalent in potatoes, fruits, vegetables, and many snack foods
- Protease—will break down proteins found in meats, nuts, eggs, and cheese
- Lipase—will break down fats found in most dairy products, nuts, oils, and meat

Without these digestive enzymes, nutrients in food can't be broken down and utilized by the body. In the case of metabolic enzymes, these are enzymes made within the cells of the body to perform specialized task required for life and health.

Enzymes work on the lock and key analogy. As you can see in the figure below, the substrate which is the food molecule, collides with the active site of the enzyme and actually attaches. The enzyme catalyzes, or breaks down, the substrate which is released in the form of the broken down molecular structure but the enzyme remains intact. Only the correct sized key (substrate) fits into the keyhole (active site) of the lock (enzyme). The lock and key analogy was first postulated in 1894 by Emil Fischer.[24]

As noted, they are specific for the food they act on, therefore an amylase cannot breakdown of protein, a protease cannot breakdown of fat, and a lipase cannot breakdown a carbohydrate.

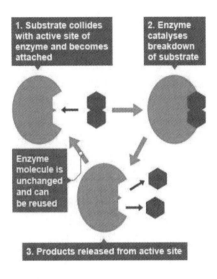

Figure 8 http://a.files.bbci.co.uk/bam/live/content/z4r2n39/small

Food enzymes are those enzymes found in raw, whole, uncooked, unprocessed foods. These enzymes are specifically matched to the composition of the food in which they are contained. For example fruits that are rich in carbohydrates contain enzymes that can break down the carbohydrates in each fruit. Fruits do not have much protein, and therefore, have very few protease enzymes for breaking down proteins. The enzyme composition of foods is designed by nature to assist in the digestion and breakdown of foods. When the enzymes are present in raw foods we eat, these foods "pre-digest" themselves and are readily assimilated and digested.

The human body was designed to function on raw, enzyme-rich foods which support the digestive and metabolic enzymes found naturally in the body. Today, much of what we eat is not real whole food loaded with beneficial enzymes. Our food usually is not fermented, therefore there are no live active enzymes. Many of us eat fruits and vegetables that are frozen, canned, or otherwise processed. It is important to remember that when foods are taken to a temperature that exceeds 118°F, live active enzymes are destroyed. Enzymes also have their own optimal pH range in which they are active. If the pH is outside this range, the enzyme will become inactive.

Consider what you get when you purchase prepackaged food. First, it has no live active enzymes. If there were live active enzymes in a prepackaged food, the food would continuously break down and rot. Knowing this, a box that sits on a store shelf for several months and then comes home and sits on your pantry shelf for several months could not possibly have live active enzymes present.

The same holds true for frozen foods. For example, if you put up your own vegetables you know that before you freeze those vegetables, you need to blanch them. This blanching requires that you put them into boiling water for a brief period of time. The purpose is to kill the live active enzymes so once the frozen food is stored, it will not rot. If you have ever tried to cut corners and skip this vital step, you have most likely had quite a mess to clean up and throw away once those foods defrosted. Yes, I know this from experience.

Now consider what happens when you eat these prepared foods, which are cooked before serving and void of all active enzymes. The enzymes' job must happen in order for those food substances to be broken down into the molecular structures necessary to do the jobs at the cellular level, but this doesn't happen.

We talked earlier about the fact that food enters the stomach and remains in the fundus of the stomach for a brief period, during which enzymes start to break down those foods. The enzyme produced by cells in the fundus is pepsin. Pepsin will begin to break down the initial bonds of protein. However, consider if you're eating pre-processed or packaged foods, not everything you've eaten is protein.

Therefore, if there are no enzymes delivered with the food, it does not break down appropriately. The food will then travel through the stomach to the first part of the small intestine inadequately broken down and now the body calls upon the pancreas to produce all the enzymes necessary to break down that food. You are not providing the pancreas with any support.

Again, the human body was designed to function on raw, enzyme-rich foods which support the digestive and metabolic enzymes produced naturally in the body. Dr. Edward Howell (the grandfather of enzyme therapy) discovered what he called "enzyme potential." Enzyme potential is understood to be the number of enzymes each of us has the ability to make in our lifetime, either digestive or metabolic. If we call upon the system to produce a lot of digestive enzymes to digest food, the body will, in turn, produce fewer metabolic enzymes.

Dr. Howell was also one of the first scientists to point to the "law of adaptive secretion of digestive enzymes." This law states that the body will adapt or change the amount of digestive enzymes it produces according to what is needed. During the time that the food is sitting in the upper portion of the stomach the body is determining how many digestive enzymes it must make to digest that food. If food enzymes do some of the work, the body doesn't have to make as many digestive enzymes and has a lot more energy for making the necessary metabolic enzymes instead.

We are born with a certain amount of enzymes in our systems. We produce both metabolic enzymes (those responsible for running every function in the body) and we produce digestive enzymes primarily in the pancreas and the liver. Over time we lower our body's enzyme level by eating enzyme-deficient foods. When enzymes that occur naturally in foods are destroyed by heating, cooking, pasteurization or processing, our bodies must compensate. The food enzymes taken in from foods we eat like the raw, organic fruits and vegetables are the most abundant and are the foundations of optimal health. When these food enzymes are not replenished on a daily basis, our body is forced to supply all of the enzymes needed to digest any cooked food. Nature's plan calls for food enzymes to help with digestion.

After years or decades of eating patterns that lack enzymes, our bodies will eventually use up their digestive enzymes or the building blocks needed to manufacture them.

What happens when we exhaust our enzyme stores because we eat only cooked or processed foods and nothing raw or live?

If we have a shortage of digestive enzymes, two things can happen and neither one of them are healthy. The body works overtime to produce the needed enzymes required to digest the food. This additional stress adversely affects the immune system and suppresses the body's ability to protect us from disease. Also, over time, our bodies become overworked, and exhaust the enzyme stores leaving us unable to make enough enzymes to properly digest the foods we take in. This will lead to symptoms of digestive issues such as belching, bloating, cramping, GERD, and perhaps diarrhea. These symptoms are not so much the result of too much HCl, but of not enough enzymes. The un-digested food begins to pollute our body which ultimately leads to increased risk of chronic disease.

This may also be a likely cause for the increase in the numbers of people with acute and chronic pancreatitis and malabsorption syndromes. If the pancreas (which is responsible for the production of digestive and metabolic enzymes) is constantly overworked, the result may be serious and lead to chronic illness and symptoms that don't fall into any specific diagnostic category. Often, without a specific diagnosis, people spend years having their symptoms treated without ever understanding the root problem, a simple lack of food enzymes. They may be given medications to treat indigestion or bloating and gas, or perhaps chronic diarrhea but will never be told to eat more raw, organic fruits and vegetables or take a digestive enzyme supplement. The pancreas will respond first to the needs presented by food entering the system. The digestive system is designed to take food and break it down into the molecular structures necessary to do the job at the cellular level. It will work to do that job, no matter what the food is. Until the food is dealt with, the production of metabolic enzymes must be put on hold. Considering the fact the SAD diet not only consists of food lacking active enzymes but also foods loaded with preservatives, the pancreas has a difficult, nearly impossible job to do.

There are some people who debate Dr. Howell's theory of enzyme potential, but if we consider the fact that we have only so much energy available to our bodies over the span of a lifetime, if we use a lot of energy for digestion, there will be less energy available to take care of other systems in our bodies.

CHAPTER 4

PUTTING OUR FOOD TO WORK
— THE SMALL INTESTINES

This is my favorite part of the GI system.

The third phase of gastric digestion is the intestinal phase. Once food leaves the stomach, it enters the small intestine, where the majority of digestion and absorption takes place.

Anatomically the small intestine is about 20 feet long, divided into three distinct portions. The *duodenum,* the first and shortest region at about 10 inches, starts at the pyloric sphincter of the stomach and merges with the *jejunum.* The jejunum is about 8 feet long and extends to the distal part of the small intestine, the *ileum,* which is about 12 feet long and joins the large intestine at the *ileocecal sphincter.*

The inside lining of the small intestine is not just a smooth surface; it consists of numerous circular folds called *plicae circulares* lined with fingerlike projections called *villi.* These villi are covered with *microvilli.* Below is a microscopic view of the villi. The action of the stomach and the gastric juices added to the digesting food creates a substance of thick, soupy consistency called *chyme.*

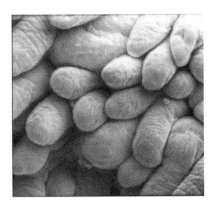

Figure 9 http://www.balanced-life-wellness.com/wp-content/uplo+ads/2011/02/villi

As chyme passes from the stomach into the first part of the small intestine, it travels through and around all these villi and microvilli, where additional chemical digestion takes place. This chemical digestion is dependent on the function of three major organs: the pancreas, the liver, and the gallbladder. The role of each will be discussed in further detail later on.

The final stages of enzymatic digestion occur here. This enzymatic activity liberates small molecules that can now be absorbed through the inside lining and picked up into the bloodstream. Special anatomical features of the inner lining, covered with villi facilitate the process of digestion and absorption.

How? First, circular mucosal folds greatly increase the small intestine's surface area. Second, by protruding into the lumen (opening), these folds aid in mixing the chyme by acting as baffles, slowing transit time through the small intestine.

The villi's fingerlike projections are covered with *epithelial* cells. In fact, this lining or membrane of fingerlike projections covered with epithelial cells, is a barrier only one cell thick. That's the only thing that separates what is outside the body from what is delivered to the inside of the body by way of digestion and absorption.

Each villus has a network of blood vessels necessary to transport the molecular structures: amino acids from proteins and simple sugars from carbohydrates, as well as a lacteal vessel that carries fats. The absorptive epithelial cells are themselves covered with microvilli as shown below.

Collectively, these features account for the huge absorptive surface area. In fact, if the small intestinal lining were removed and the villi laid flat, end to end and side to side the absorptive surface available would be about the size of a tennis court.[25] The working of this incredible factory allows nutrients to be absorbed by the epithelial cells covering the villi and passing through the walls of the capillary membrane to enter either the blood or the lymph system.

If that's not a big enough job, this membrane is also responsible as a gatekeeper. This function, when all is working properly, ensures only good things enter into the bloodstream and toxins do not.

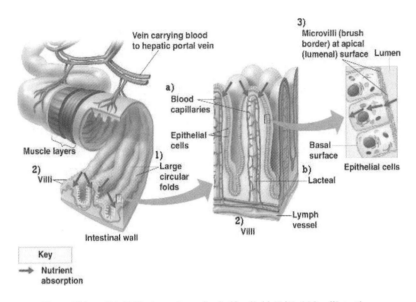

*Figure 10 http://bio1152.nicerweb.com/Locked/media/ch41/41_23SmallIntestine
Struct_L.jpg*

Intestinal juices are slightly alkaline, with an ideal pH usually around 7.6. Together these intestinal juices, pancreatic juice (delivered to the small intestine via two pancreatic ducts), and bile from the liver and gallbladder (delivered via the hepatic duct and the bile duct respectively—see figure 11) come into contact with the chyme. Now the work begins.

This mixing provides for the continual breaking down of substances in the chyme. This dynamic process usually takes 3 to 5 hours and culminates in the breaking down of the food substances particle by particle completing the digestion and absorption of carbohydrates, proteins, and fats.

The Accessory Organs of Digestion

The Pancreas

The pancreas is a gland about six to ten inches long consisting of a head, a body, and a tail. The pancreas is connected to the duodenum by two ducts (seen in figure 11). The pancreas is made up of small clusters of glandular epithelial cells. It mainly produces two types of substances: digestive juices or enzymes and hormones. Often when I mention the pancreas, people understand that it is the organ responsible for insulin production. The interesting thing is only about one percent of the cells of the pancreas are responsible for the production of insulin. These cells are organized into clusters called *pancreatic islets* (the islets of Langerhans) and this makes up the endocrine portion of the pancreas. These islet cells secrete the hormones *glucagon, insulin, somatostatin,* and *pancreatic polypeptide.*

Approximately 99 percent of the cells of the pancreas are arranged in clusters called *acini.* The cells within acini secrete a mixture of fluid and digestive enzymes called *pancreatic juice* which constitutes the exocrine (secreting substance via a duct) function of the pancreas. Sodium bicarbonate in this pancreatic juice makes it slightly alkaline (pH 7.1 to 8.2) to help neutralize the acidity of the chyme as it leave the stomach. The enzymes in this pancreatic juice include *pancreatic amylase, trypsin, chymotrypsin, carboxypeptidase, elastase,* and the principal triglyceride-digesting enzyme in adults called *pancreatic lipase*. The hormone *cholecystokinin* (CCK) is the principal stimulus for delivery of pancreatic enzymes into the small intestine. These enzymes travel through the pancreatic ducts and assist in breaking down food molecules. Food enzymes break down food molecules, digestive enzymes break down food molecules, and these pancreatic enzymes also do that job.

I cannot stress enough the importance of enzymes. I have studied this particular topic for years and find it so extremely fascinating. When we talk about enzymes and, in particular, the pancreatic enzymes, in his book *Enzymes: The Key to Health*, Dr. Howard Loomis, Jr. also discusses the fact every person is born with an enzyme potential. As noted earlier, this is explained as the number of enzymes a person can produce in a lifetime. This number is determined by the DNA code. In addition, each enzyme can only perform a certain amount of work before it becomes exhausted and must be replaced by another. Along with digesting processed food, enzyme supply can be diminished by caffeinated and alcoholic beverages, colds and fevers, stress pregnancy, strenuous exercise, injuries, and extreme weather conditions. [26]

Dr. Howell's "Enzyme Nutrition Axiom" pretty well says it all. "The length of life is inversely proportional to the rate of exhaustion of the enzyme potential of an organism."[27] The understanding is a shortened lifespan, inferior health of the organs, and nagging illnesses all due to an enzyme-deficient diet.

If we do not eat an enzyme-rich diet, we deplete our enzyme potential without replenishing it. This is why eating some uncooked organic fruits and vegetables—or drinking the juice of those same fruits and vegetables, along with enzyme supplementation—is essential. Juicing is actually very beneficial because once you have juiced fresh, organic fruits and vegetables, you are left with a liquid, abundant with enzymes, that doesn't have to be broken down in the stomach in order for those enzymes to be released.

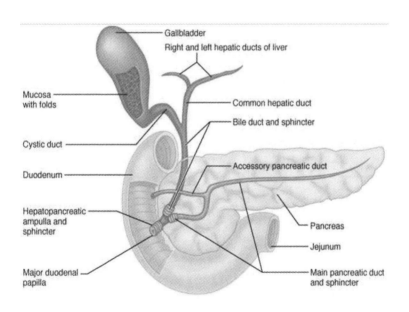

Figure 11 http://apbrwww5.apsu.edu/thompsonj/Anatomy%20&%20Physiology/2020/2020%20Exam%20Reviews/Exam%203/Pancreas%20diagram

The Liver
—*The Metabolic Warehouse of the Body*

At three pounds, the liver weighs in as the heaviest gland in the body. It is divided into two principal lobes, with the larger lobe on the right. The liver is often referred to as the metabolic warehouse of the body. Here detoxification takes place as discussed below. In addition, worn-out white blood cells, red blood cells, bacteria, and other foreign matter that drains through veins from the gastrointestinal (GI) tract are destroyed. Because blood that leaves the GI tract passes through the liver, it is often the site for metastasis of cancer originating in the GI tract.

In addition to detoxification, the liver plays a critical role in our body's ability to digest and absorb fats. The liver is responsible for the production of bile, and the human adult produces 400 to 800 ml of bile a day. Bile is a green, brown, or yellow liquid which has a pH of 7.6 to 8.6. It consists mostly of water, bile acids, bile salts, a phospholipid (a fatty compound) called lecithin, cholesterol, bile pigments, and several ions or electrically charged atoms. The role of bile is to emulsify large fat globules breaking them into smaller globules. Just as dish detergent works breaking up large globules of fat into smaller globules while washing dishes, bile does the same thing to fats in the body. Many waste products are eliminated from the body by secretion into the bile and, ultimately, elimination in the feces. Hepatic synthesis of bile acids accounts for the majority of cholesterol breakdown in the body. In humans approximately 500 mg of cholesterol are converted into bile acids and eliminated in bile every day.[28]

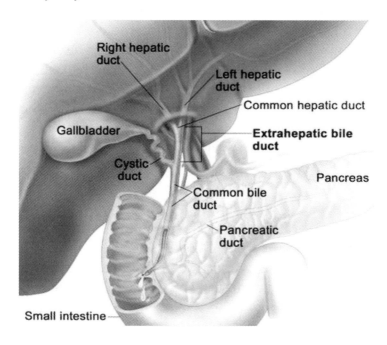

Figure 12
https://images.duckduckgo.com/iu/?u=http%3A%2F%2Fwww.uchospitals.edu%2Fim ages%2Fnci%2FCDR0000658899.jpg&f=1

As for the detoxification function of the liver, it is one of four major organs that eliminate toxins. These toxins come from internal sources while we're breaking down the foods that we eat. They enter through the cell membranes of the gastrointestinal tract. Toxins also come from external sources, entering through the cell membranes of our skin and lungs. External toxins come from the perfumes, hairspray, body lotions, body wash, shaving cream, toothpaste, etc. before we even leave the bathroom in the morning.

Then if we eat the SAD diet, perhaps a couple of toaster waffles and coffee with artificial flavoring, we introduce more toxins. The liver filters the blood to remove large toxins; synthesizes and gets rid of bile full of cholesterol and other fat-soluble toxins; and enzymatically eliminates unwanted chemicals. During this process, free radicals are produced. Too many free radicals can damage liver cells.[29]

The liver is responsible for many other functions such as carbohydrate and protein metabolism, the excretion of bilirubin, and the storage of glycogen, vitamins A, B 12, D, E, and K as well as minerals and trace minerals. It is responsible for *phagocytosis,* which is the process whereby cells can engulf and subsequently ingest particles of bacteria. The liver also activates vitamin D. One other very important role, or function, of the liver is the processing and regulation of hormone function. Knowing the liver is responsible for so many functions, I have to now revisit the GMO issue.

I talked earlier about GM foods and glyphosate. The study in *Entropy* I referenced was an extensive, systematic researching of the literature on the part of the authors. This revealed several interesting facts ultimately linking glyphosate use to many diseases that are on the rise.

One of the main findings of the report is that glyphosate inhibits *cytochrome P450* (CYP) enzyme production in the liver. These enzymes are a diverse, ancient class of enzymes that date back three billion years and play an important role in plant, animal, and microbial biology. These enzymes have a role in: metabolism of drugs, foreign chemicals, cholesterol metabolism and bile-acid biosynthesis; steroid synthesis and metabolism; vitamin D (3) synthesis; and metabolism. We know the liver does all these things. Cytochrome P450 was once believed to be mainly a hepatic drug detox-ification system, but is now understood to include a myriad of enzymatic liver reactions implicated in important life processes. Mutations in many CYP genes cause inborn errors of metabolism and contribute to many clinically relevant diseases.[30]

One of the functions of CYP enzymes is to detoxify *xenobiotics*, chemical compounds found in living organisms that are not normally produced or consumed by the organism. Healthy CYP enzyme function includes the cleaning up of these chemical compounds that are destructive to organs and tissues throughout the body. By limiting the ability of these enzymes to detoxify foreign chemical compounds, glyphosate, the active ingredient in Roundup not only interferes with the function of healthy gut bacteria but actually *exaggerates* the damaging effects of any chemicals and environ-mental toxins we are exposed to. It just is not safe for human consumption.

You may not consider drinking Roundup but it gets inside you any time you eat GM foods or their byproducts that have been grown in the fields sprayed with Roundup. It is interesting to note the use of Roundup is increasing as the weeds have begun to outsmart the Roundup and continue to grow despite being sprayed. More and more is necessary to have the desired killing effect so more is pulled up by the plants as they grow. It makes me wonder what new chemical they'll come up with to kill weeds. What ill effects will new chemicals have on the human body?

Many of the specific functions of the liver are known to be regulated by the CYP enzymes. They are necessary for the formation of water-soluble bile acids from cholesterol to emulsify and hydrolyze (break apart using water) fats. Both cholesterol and vitamin D3 synthesis and degradation depend upon various CYP enzymes. Two CYP enzymes in the liver catalyze (speed up reactions) 25–hydroxylation of vitamin D3 to its active form, and two other CYP enzymes catalyze the breakdown of vitamin D3 in the liver.[31]

What does all of this mean? It means the CYP enzymes, like all enzymes are very fascinating, busy little proteins. They are essential for various reactions to occur and are critical to many functions of the liver. Forming the water-soluble (dissolve in water) bile is necessary to ensure the breakdown of fats in our foods. This is so the body can absorb and utilize essential fatty acids and the fat soluble vitamins. The imbalance created by the interruption of these reactions affect both liver and gallbladder function. Could this be part of the reason we are removing sick gallbladders from teenagers? They are eating too many GMO foods.

These various chemical reactions take place continually in the liver and these reactions are regulated by these CYP enzymes. As described above, Vitamin D cannot be properly manufactured or regulated by the liver if these CYP enzymes don't function properly. Could this be part of the reason so many suffer from Vitamin D deficiency?

Several CYP enzymes participate in steroid synthesis (the production of steroids). Five crucial hormones, *aldosterone, androstenedione, cortisol, corticosterone, and dehydroepiandrosterone* (DHEA0029x, are produced in the adrenal glands, testes and ovaries, and in the adrenal cortex. These are called steroid hormones and all steroid hormones are produced from cholesterol by reactions requiring these CYP enzymes. The lipophilic (promoting the dissolvability of fats) nature of these steroids allows them to diffuse across fatty membranes to get the job done. A specific CYP enzyme, CYP19A1 (aromatase), whose inhibition has been confirmed in association with glyphosate, converts androgenic precursors into estrogen.[32] This creates a hormonal imbalance. Hormone regulation, a very important part of live function is interfered with if CYP enzyme production is inhibited due to glyphosate. Could this be part of the reason so many men and women have this problem? Could this be why the symptoms of menopause and andropause (male menopause) plague us like never before? Could this be part of the reason why so many are struggling to get pregnant? We are human beings and procreation should not be this difficult! We are human beings and going through "the change" should not be a crisis!

In summary: glyphosate's dramatic, impact on the liver's ability to function normally and in a healthy way is clearly shown in these studies. Considering these functions, the liver controls detoxification, vitamin D activation, and hormone regulation to name a few, combined with the fact glyphosate has such a profound effect on the function of the CYP enzymes regulating these processes and the healthy function of the liver, our metabolic warehouse, I must conclude, the use of glyphosate on crops, with resulting human ingestion of glyphosate while consuming GM foods, has contributed greatly to more and more people plagued with chronic disease and infertility.

The Gallbladder
—Not Without My Gallbladder

The gallbladder is a 3- to 4-inch pear-shaped sac located in a depression of the rear surface of the liver (seen in the picture above). The primary function of the gallbladder is to: 1) receive bile produced by the liver; and 2) act as a receptacle to store that bile, so that ample amounts are readily available to ensure the emulsification and proper digestion of fats. The presence of fat in the duodenum is the most potent stimulus for the release of cholecystokinin (CCK), which stimulates the contraction of the gallbladder's wall, to squeeze out the stored bile. This concentrated bile is mixed with mineral salts and enzymes that are released into the first part of the small intestine, the duodenum. Malfunction of the gallbladder will result in impairment of fat digestion and absorption.

It is not uncommon to see people with gallbladder disease. In my experience I've seen many people, some as young as late teens and early 20s, present with the typical signs of gallbladder issues. They describe right epigastric pain, up under the ribs on the right side of the upper abdomen, sometimes severe, sometimes a stabbing pain in the chest, sometimes a stabbing pain between the shoulder blades, sometimes a feeling of a tight band wrapped around the chest, and all related to having consumed a fatty meal.

Perhaps they've had pizza or ice cream, both of which would call on the gallbladder to produce the bile necessary to break down the fats. If the gallbladder is full of sludge or stones, it may not release adequate amounts of bile, thus bringing on these physical symptoms. People may also describe fatty diarrhea, nausea, vomiting, and general malaise.

Conventional medicine's approach to this is to quickly do an ultrasound to determine if, in fact, it is the gallbladder. Once the ultrasound confirms the gallbladder is full of sludge or stones, the person is admitted to the hospital and put on the surgery schedule so the gallbladder can be removed promptly the next day. I have seen it done many times and was even "privileged" to have it happen to me.

On three separate occasions I experienced the horrible pain scenario. The first time I really didn't know what it was. It was associated with nausea and some vomiting, so I suspected I had eaten something that disagreed with me. The second time I found myself wondering what I had done that was similar to the first episode, and realized I had eaten pizza both times. Certainly the cheese on the pizza, loaded with fat, could have been a contributor.

During the third episode, I was scheduled to lecture the next morning and was overcome with excruciating pain and symptoms even more profound than the prior two events. I ended up in the emergency room. All the standard testing was done, even a pregnancy test (certainly not necessary at my age having experienced the thrill of menopause several years earlier) protocol because I am female! Really? Is it any wonder our healthcare and medical insurance systems are so costly and in such a mess? The ultrasound revealed that I had some large stones in my gallbladder, and of course I would be admitted and meet with the surgeon in the morning so my gallbladder could be removed. Well, that wasn't going to happen because I had to speak the next day. So after the very caring nurse, concerned physician's assistant, and overwhelmed emergency room physician all took their turn trying to convince me I needed to go through with the surgery, I signed out Against Medical Advice (AMA), assuring them I knew what to do and how to handle my issue. Fortunately I was given a prescription for pain medicine that allowed me to sleep that night and speak on Saturday.

The following day, Sunday, bright and early, I started my standard liver/gallbladder flush. Although I was very sick and the pain was relentless, I managed to make it through that night and on Monday saw the evidence of the ER staff's concern through the passing of large, fat globules and large stones.

I did not want to lose my gallbladder. I know that many people live very happily without a gallbladder and have no more symptoms. I have also worked with several individuals who have had their gallbladders removed, and continued to have the same symptoms they had before the surgery was done. I've always believed if your gallbladder is not working properly, removing it won't make it work any better. People who have had their gallbladders removed may tell me they have no symptoms, but I know removal can lead to long-term problems with fatty acid absorption and assimilation of the fat-soluble vitamins A, D, E, and K.

Several years prior to my event, I had learned about liver/gallbladder flushing and had decided it sounded like a healthy thing to do from an all-natural health perspective, so I tried it. I remember researching the process and finding pictures on the Internet of little green jellybeans that I would ultimately see in the toilet. I told myself I would not see little green jellybeans in the toilet, yet I did. The thing I found most interesting was I had never had a symptom before that time. Even more interesting, I never had a symptom while I passed all the stones. I repeated the process about eight weeks later, and had another very good result passing stones. Before this happened I had done that liver/gallbladder flush periodically, at least twice a year.

So what happened? Why was I stricken with such a sick gallbladder? I actually had to do some research to find the answer, but am convinced I know now what happened. I had been on a very strict weight-releasing program, losing a significant amount of body weight and, subsequently, fat. This program included a very low-fat diet. These two things, rapid weight loss and a low-fat diet, were major contributors.

During this research I learned that while my liver was processing all the released fat, it was forcing more cholesterol than usual into my gallbladder. In addition, my low-fat diet did not call on the gallbladder to pump out the usual necessary bile. This actually threw my gallbladder into a situation of imbalance. This accumulation of cholesterol allowed crystals to precipitate out and stones began to develop. I had my answer. I can also relate to anyone who has the pain associated with gallbladder problems. I am compassionate by nature but more so when it comes to gallbladder pain. I remember being asked to rate my pain and telling them it was every bit as bad as the pain I experienced giving birth.

CHAPTER 5

THE ROLE OF THE DIGESTIVE SYSTEM IN OVERALL HEALTH AND IMMUNITY

This is beyond digestion and absorption of nutrients.

Gut Bacteria

When I talk about gut bacteria, I'm talking about *probiotics*, also known as healthy gut flora or gut microbiota. Examples are beneficial bacteria like the *Lactobacillus* and *Bifidobacterium* strains determined necessary to keep us healthy and our digestive systems in balance.

The term probiotics was first used in 1965 to describe microorganisms that confer very beneficial properties on other microorganisms. Since that time, research into probiotics and their health implications has been extensive. The term probiotics has evolved to incorporate any organism that has beneficial impact on another organism.

The word probiotic is a combination of two words of Greek origin. *Pro* signifies "the promotion of" and *biotic* means "life," hence "the promotion of life." Let's take a minute to define the human gut *microbiome*. First, understand this field of study is still so new, there is no firm and agreed-upon definition. The American Academy of Microbiology, an honorific branch of the American Society of Microbiology, should have a pretty good idea of the definition. Its publication *Human Microbiome FAQ* states that microbiome has two definitions: one genetic and one ecological.

> Definition 1: Just as the entire collection of human genes is called the human genome, this definition of microbiome means the entire collection of genes found in all of the microbes associated with a particular host. A broader term, "metagenome," means the entire collection of microbial genes found in a particular environment. A "metagenome" may or may not be host-associated—metagenomes have been generated for sea water, shower-heads, and hot springs, among many other environments.

> Definition 2: Ecologists use the term "biome" to describe the collection of plants and animals that live in a particular environment. Thus there are various terrestrial and aquatic biomes (temperate grasslands, or tropical coral reefs, for example) that are characterized by similar climatic conditions and collections of organisms. When microbiome is used in this sense, it

refers to the ecosystem made up of microbes within and on the human body—that is, the collection of microbes that live in the human habitat.[33]

Now, let's sort that all out. First, gut microbiota was formerly known as gut flora. Many of us still call it flora, referring to healthy or friendly gut flora vs. unhealthy gut flora (not always unhealthy, but labeled that because overgrowth of the "less than desirable" microbes is often problematic). As human organisms we have lots of flora/microbes that are part of who we are. These microbes are bacteria, fungi, viruses, etc. that live on us and in us, on our skin, in our mouths, in the respiratory system, in the vagina, and in the digestive system.

In fact, in the human digestive system (or gut, as I most often call it), we have tens of trillions of microorganisms. It is estimated at least 500 to 1,000 different species are present in the gut.[34] These bacteria outnumber our cells by about 10 to 1.[35] That's a lot of bacteria. So some are very beneficial, actually necessary; others cause problems if allowed to overgrow. The important thing is they must be kept in balance. If we have too many of the "unhealthy," as we refer to them, and not enough of the friendly, we get into trouble. In the human gut, the microbiome directly influences biochemical, physiological and immunological pathways and is the first line of resistance to various diseases.[36]

OK, so why do we call the less than desirable microbes unhealthy? More accurately, how do they get that way? *Candida* is a type of yeast that is part of us. It is commonly found in the mucous membranes; the mouth, gut, urinary tract, and vagina. As a yeast, *Candida* resides in the small intestine right there with the lactobacilli (one of the friendly bacteria). These two are the predominant residents of the small intestine (not the large intestine or colon as is often suggested). These two bacteria are content to cohabitate, if you will, until or unless the *Candida* gets angry and transforms from a yeast to a fungus. This happens due to an imbalance, and the resultant proliferation or overgrowth cause problems. In the transformation *Candida* goes from being a *dimorphic* organism, meaning it is a round yeast cell, to being a fungus with spindly outgrowths called *hyphae.* These hyphae can penetrate the body tissue and cause a breakdown in the integrity of the wall of the intestine, the villi and microvilli, leading to what we know as "leaky gut syndrome."

One of the easiest ways to understand leaky gut is to think about a window screen. If that window screen is intact, only tiny little bugs can get through the holes. If that screen is not intact and has larger holes in it, larger bugs can get through those holes. A similar thing is happening in the gut. Those little microscopic holes, created by tight junctions in the lining of the small intestines, allow tiny nutrient molecules to pass through and into the bloodstream. This is the normal process. Larger holes, created by inflammation of the intestinal lining and the break-down and loosening of these junctions allow larger than normal nutrient molecules, especially protein molecules, to cross and get picked up into the bloodstream. This is not normal. This is leaky gut.

If you are healthy, your gut is healthy, and you have ample amounts of lactobacilli bacteria, *Candida* overgrowth is not a problem. *Candida* is kept in check by the friendly bacteria and remains a harmless yeast. Living in harmony or symbiosis, the *Candida* behaves itself, if you will, and the good friendly bacteria help keep us well. Healthy bacteria like the lactobacilli are responsible for several things:

- Better absorption of foods because of the enzymes they produce
- Increase in peristalsis (wave of contraction that moves food through the intestine) helping to normalize bowel movements
- Increase in immunity through the secretion of acids and natural antibiotics
- Maintenance of good hormonal balance
- Vitamin production, especially the B vitamins
- Stabilization and balancing of cholesterol levels
- Defending against foodborne illness
- Keeping the intestinal walls fed by creating short-chain fatty acids

At birth these bacteria/microflora begin to colonize our guts. During birth, the baby is exposed to bacteria coming through the vaginal canal. These begin to colonize the gut immediately. If a child is born caesarean section, colonization is in part due to the mother's microflora, but is more likely from the birthing environment, staff, or other babies while in the nursery. For this reason, C-section babies don't have the same microflora benefits and may suffer from excessive colic, diarrhea, and constipation. This happens because soon after birth *Candida* must be balanced with approximately 85 percent good bacteria to the 15 percent yeast-type bacteria. If left "unguarded," the *Candida* may be encouraged to change its structure to the unfriendly fungal form.

Friendly bacteria are necessary to stimulate the growth of the intestinal lining and the immune system in the intestine. They prevent the over-growth of other disease-causing bacteria within the intestine. Friendly bacteria produce vitamin K, which is absorbed and used by the host. These bacteria are also important for the muscular activity of the small intestine. Without friendly bacteria, there is reduced muscular activity, therefore reduced peristalsis.

As we age, the levels of friendly bacteria will lessen over time. We are also exposed to a number of irritants each day that severely diminish the friendly bacteria. This creates an imbalance of the healthy gut environment or a *dysbiosis*, the opposite of *symbiosis* (organisms living together in harmony). The worst culprits are:

- Antibiotics and steroids—medicines we take as well as those injected into livestock

- Chlorinated water—in the form of tap water or exposure when we take a shower
- Antacids and or anti-inflammatory drugs
- Stress—acute as well as chronic
- Radiation, chemotherapy, x-rays
- Caffeine, tobacco, and alcohol
- Prescription and over–the–counter medications
- The Standard American Diet—SAD diet

Let's consider some of these culprits in more detail.

When you take an antibiotic, it is generally prescribed to kill a bacterial infection. Well, it will also kill the healthy bacteria in the gut, creating that imbalance that allows for a proliferation of the fungal form of yeast-type bacteria.

Obviously, water is very important and we should drink plenty each day. However, if you're drinking tap water, most tap water coming through a city water treatment plant has been treated with chlorine. Drinking chlorine will, of course, kill the healthy bacteria in your gut. Taking a shower in chlorinated water is even more harmful. You actually inhale chloroform, a byproduct of chlorine, while taking a shower or a hot bath. Research has demonstrated that the amount you breathe in—and what your skin absorbs while taking a 10-minute shower—is greater than the amount you would ingest drinking eight glasses of water.[37]

Antacids decrease the amount of acid in the stomach. This lower digestive acid secretion promotes the yeast overgrowth. Anti-inflammatories, especially nonsteroidal anti-inflammatories (called NSAIDs like Motrin, Aleve, and Ibuprofen) actually cause a leaky gut because they inflame the inside lining of the gut, creating a widening of the spaces between the cells (puts larger holes in the screen). Apart from antibiotics, they are the second largest group of drugs to cause or aggravate leaky gut syndrome (LGS).[38] NSAIDs are said to slow down and eventually block the enzyme that produces *prostaglandins*. Prostaglandins (lipid compounds that have hormone messenger-like effects) modulate inflammation. NSAIDs block the prostaglandins that stimulate tissue repair in the body, as well as the ones that cause pain. They may temporarily inhibit pain in some parts of the body, but they do increase intestinal permeability. They are damaging to the microvilli in the intestine, causing allergies and eventually making pain in the other parts of the body worse as well. The damaged intestine cannot repair because the NSAIDs have blocked the production of the prostaglandins that heal tissues. Among patients who chronically use NSAIDs, research has suggested that 65 percent will develop intestinal inflammation.[39]

Acute and chronic stress will predispose a person to illness and disease. We all know people who are stressed. There is a considerable amount of research being done to help better understand this connection. Research demonstrates a healthy gut microbiome not only affects the gut and the immune system, but also the mind. The gut is often referred to as the "second brain." It is the only organ that has its own independent nervous system, an intricate network of 100 million neurons embedded in the gut wall. This neural network is so sophisticated, the gut continues to function even when the primary neural conduit between it and the brain, the vagus nerve, is severed.[40]

About 80 to 90 percent of the neurotransmitter serotonin is produced with in the gastrointestinal tract—*not* the brain. Since large quantities of neurotransmitters are manufactured in the gut, this means your GI tract is largely responsible for your general physical *and* mental wellbeing.[41] Any stress, acute or chronic from any cause affects the microbiome, and an unhealthy microbiome affects how the body responds to stress. There is currently much research into the gut-brain connection and the link between an unhealthy gut microbiome and conditions like brain fog, depression, autism, Alzheimer's, social anxiety, ADD/ADHD, and so on. I will go into much more detail about this exciting topic in my next book.

Traveling is an example of an environmental stressor causing changes in our normal microbiome composition, or its gene expression (when the genes are copied into our RNA). This may lead to transient (as in travelers' diarrhea) or permanent dominance of pathogenic gut bacteria.[42]

Also, a recent study demonstrated that exposure to a social stressor altered the composition of the intestinal microbiome in mice, indicating stressor-induced immunomodulation. It was demonstrated that stressor exposure changes the stability of the microflora and leads to bacterial translocation (leaving the intestinal tract and entering the blood stream or lymphatic system).[43] So, the immune system was compromised and changes in the stability of the microflora allowed toxins to leak out of the intestine and into the body. This was all caused by exposure to a social stressor. Wow!

Caffeine and tobacco kill off friendly bacteria. Now am I going to tell you to stop drinking coffee? That would be pretty hypocritical on my part, as I drink coffee. I enjoy one to two cups a day, and do not consume much other caffeine beyond that. I realize that the caffeine will kill off the healthy bacteria, so I make sure I replenish each day with a good probiotic product. As for smoking, I'm not going to tell you that's OK. I believe smoking causes far too much damage from many other perspectives. Alcohol, on occasion and in moderation, is probably not harmful. Be aware when people consume alcohol on a daily basis they are killing off the friendly bacteria and further injuring the inside lining of the intestines, among many other things.

Most prescription and over-the-counter (OTC) drugs will kill off the friendly bacteria. The list is long. Antibiotics, NSAIDs, birth control pills, steroids, and other drugs interfere with stomach acid production and irritate the intestinal lining.

It should go without saying that the SAD diet impacts friendly bacteria. Large amounts of sugar, fried foods, preservatives, GMO, high-fructose corn syrup, the list goes on and on. These foods may contain pesticide residues and other poisons. Pre-packaged and processed foods often contain up to 100 chemical additives. These chemicals include flavorings, preservatives, dough conditioners, artificial and natural sweeteners, MSG, aspartame, and literally hundreds of others. The result is *Candida* overgrowth. Remember, now those *Candida* yeast have turned into the ugly fungal form. There is not enough friendly bacteria; therefore dysbiosis exists. Symptoms range from subtle and hardly noticeable to profound, interfering with an active lifestyle.

Some of the symptoms of dysbiosis are:

- Fatigue—often chronic often most noticeable after eating
- Poor digestion, constipation, diarrhea, gas, bloating, cramps, heartburn
- Foul-smelling breath, foul-smelling stools
- Vaginal infections, impotence, rectal itch, urinary infections, prostatitis
- Skin irritations like eczema, hives, psoriasis, athlete's foot, jock itch
- Frequent colds and flu, postnasal drip, bronchitis, asthma, sore throats
- Allergies, to food and airborne chemicals
- Sugar cravings, mood swings, headaches (especially migraines), poor concentration, dizziness, depression and anxiety, brain fog, ADD, ADHD
- In early childhood—hyperactivity, excessive anger, cradle cap, rashes, thrush, chronic infections

When you look at this long list you may think, wow, really? The answer is yes, really. The digestive system is very closely linked to your body's overall immune system. In fact, there is a very strong link between gut health and the immune system. Approximately 70 to 80 percent of your immune tissue is located within your digestive system. The gut is often the first entry point for exposure to pathogens (bad bacteria and viruses that can cause disease), so your gut immune system must be thriving and healthy to keep you healthy and avoid illness. The gut is a large interface between the outside world and the internal environment. From the mouth to anus, the digestive system constitutes the body's second largest surface area. The intestinal mucosa provides a dual the role in that it provides a barrier which, if healthy and intact, prohibits macromolecules and microbes from entering the systemic circulation while absorbing critical nutrients. Simply said, if your gut isn't healthy, you're not healthy.

A Personal Story

This relationship and impact between good gut health and immunity was clearly demonstrated to me many years ago. In fact, the story I'm about to share is what drove my passion to help other people understand the impact of good digestive health.

When my son was two years old (he's now 22 and not fond of me telling this story), he developed a bad ear infection and strep throat. It took three rounds of antibiotics to kill the infection. During the third course of antibiotics, he developed a horrible diarrhea and became very dehydrated. His little eyes were sunken with big dark circles around them, and he looked horribly sick. At that time, I knew enough to recognize that we had killed off his good healthy bacteria, and I went to the pharmacy and was able to get *Lactobacillus acidophilus*. After starting this regimen, within 24 hours my son's diarrhea subsided and he was much improved. However, within a few short weeks, he developed horrible eczema. This was not a mild case of eczema. It was down his back, across his bum, behind his knees, in the bends of his arms, under his arms, and across his scalp.

As a caring mom, I took him to his pediatrician. The only suggestion offered was a course of steroids. Well, I knew enough about steroids to be very concerned. I knew he already had a problem with his immune system due to the issue at hand. Understanding the impact of steroid therapy on adrenal function, I simply said, no. From time to time we would use mild steroid creams when the condition got out of hand, as it often did. For eight years he lived with this condition. It was recognized he had lactose intolerance, because if he consumed dairy products like ice cream or cheese, he would have what I call a "flare" where his eczema would become very weepy and more irritated. So he ate very little in terms of dairy. Recognizing wheat as a potential allergen, he ate very little of that, although we never did observe an obvious link between wheat consumption and the eczema flares. We tried oatmeal baths, we tried lotions, we tried creams, we tried everything topically I could possibly find with only minimal improvement. We started taking high quality nutritional supplementation. The eczema got better, but never really went away. We increased his essential fatty acids and it improved, but again, never went away.

One afternoon I had occasion to discuss his issues with two naturopathic friends. Their questioning went along the lines of whether or not he had ever had a course of antibiotics, to which I shared the story and told them that I had given him *Lactobacillus acidophilus*. The response was that I had only done part of the job. In fact, I needed to give him more strains of probiotic and be more strict with his diet, especially with dairy and wheat. Well, at the age of 10, I sat him down and told him no dairy and no wheat. Of course his response was, "Ma, what am I going to eat?" I told him we would try this for a couple of weeks and if we did not see a marked improvement, we would continue to look for the answer.

As God is my witness, within three days his eczema was so much better I couldn't believe it. Within five days it was gone. The eczema he had lived with for eight years was literally gone. I was amazed! How could probiotics fix this problem so quickly? At this point I began my ongoing research which has led to my understanding and knowledge of probiotics and good gut health.

Interesting things that I learned and observed in my son were not only did the eczema clear up; he no longer had lactose intolerance. It did not matter if he ate ice cream or cheese, these things did not bother him and caused no evidence of eczema. About six years after his recovery, we were on vacation and, although he had been very healthy up until that time, he was worn down by late night study for exams and trying to get ready for spring break. His immune system wavered and he developed a bad strep throat. I was able to get a course of antibiotics and, within 24 hours of starting his antibiotic, we were already seeing evidence of eczema. He looked at me and simply said, "Ma, don't worry about it; as soon as we are home I'll start my probiotics."

Upon our return home, he started his probiotics and digestive enzymes and within 24 hours his eczema was clearing and within three days was completely gone again. This experience made a believer out of me. If the simple act of cleaning up the diet, taking probiotics and digestive enzymes on top of all the healthy nutrition he was already taking was all it took to clear up the eczema, I wanted the world to know.

In sharing this message with all who will listen and with much research and study on my part, I have helped many people conquer conditions related to an unhealthy gut. Allergies, autoimmune diseases, fibromyalgia, chronic fatigue syndrome, rheumatoid arthritis, lupus, depression, the list goes on and on. The human body is a fantastic healing machine and if you give it the raw materials it needs, and ensure that you are putting only healthy nutrients into the precious internal environment while periodically cleaning out the detox pathways, you will be much healthier and, of course, happier.

Allergies

People often come to me with concerns about allergies. My first response is always to recommend cleaning up the gut.

An important role of the immune system is to distinguish self from non-self. Put another way, distinguish foreign molecules from the molecules that make up the tissues within our bodies. The digestive system is made up of cells, proteins, tissues, and organs all working together to defend the body against harmful bacteria, infectious diseases, and toxins. The immune system responds to foreign molecules by multiplying specialized white blood cells (*lymphocytes*) and by producing antibodies. The gut mucosa or lining connects with the largest population of immune cells in the body. These are known as gastrointestinal immune cells, which come from a special part of the immune system. The secretion of these special cells sets up the attack on harmful invaders. These lymphocyte cells work to protect the mucous membranes of the small intestines from infection. They release specific white blood cells known as T cells and B cells that defend the inside of the digestive tract from infection, as well as the damage harmful bacteria and toxins cause to the intestinal walls.

As mentioned before, everything must be in balance. When the intestinal wall begins to lose integrity because of a variety of chemically mediated conditions and the imbalance of friendly and unfriendly bacteria, the tight junctions become loose junctions and the membrane becomes permeable (those large holes in the screen). Now, larger-than-normal sized food molecules leak into the circulation.

When this occurs, the immune system kicks into high gear. These large food molecules are seen as foreign invaders and the immune system mounts an attack. The liver gets involved trying to clean up the toxins, but it becomes overwhelmed. Toxins then re-enter the circulation. The circulatory system becomes overwhelmed and can't effectively deal with all the toxins, which eventually become deposited in the muscle tissue and the joints creating a myriad of symptoms, many of which are not well understood. The reason for this is the mechanism by which they are deposited in the first place, is not well understood.

This is all happening as a result of the immune system trying to do its job. When a foreign invader is first recognized, special immune cells (called *dendritic* cells) discover the culprit, snatch a piece, and present it to other special immune cells called T cells. Simplistically, the antigen (culprit) is delivered to the T cell and the resulting cascade of events sets the remainder of the immune system response in motion.[44] The body now responds with inflammation, allergies, and symptoms related to a very long list of diseases conventional medicine will see and treat, repeatedly, often with little success because the symptoms are being treated but not the root cause. These long-term, often debilitating, and life-threatening diseases are placed into the category known as autoimmune.

Autoimmune Disorders/Diseases

While working as a nutritional support nurse back in the early 1980s, I clearly remember attending conferences addressing health concerns and the challenges faced by people who could no longer eat by mouth, as well as those in the general population. At that time chronic fatigue and fibromyalgia were both spoken of, but because neither was well understood or specifically related to the gut, most people with the vague complaints associated with these conditions were looked upon as perhaps just a little "crazy." These complaints had not been seen in such large numbers of people before now, yet they were the topic of presentations.

Because conventional medicine could not come up with a diagnosis and had no "cure," if you presented with these symptoms, you would likely be told "It's all in your head." Many were referred to psychologists and psychiatrists; perhaps the stress of everyday life was just too much. Many were given antidepressants and sleeping pills to help with their unusual symptoms. These conditions were given names, they were increasingly diagnosed, and pharmaceutical companies got to work and made millions creating specific drugs to treat the specific conditions. We certainly have come a long way since that time. Although you're not likely to get anything other than a drug from a conventional physician, naturopaths and functional medicine doctors recognize what's going on, and many understand it is most often related to an unhealthy gut.

It's interesting that these conditions have become so prevalent. When we consider some of the causal factors, starting at the very beginning with the foods we eat and all the issues previously mentioned, it really isn't difficult to understand why we are seeing so many people sick with these conditions.

If the gut wall is permeable and the partially undigested food, bacteria, toxins and viruses are passing through and stimulating a chronic immune system response, problems are going to happen. The immune system will become overwhelmed. We now have inflammatory triggers circulating throughout the circulatory system.

The inflammatory response is normal and occurs when there is any type of damage or injury to a tissue, organ, or structure within the body. Imagine banging your shin. It's not long before the inflammatory response is in full force. You now have a lump, it's red, it's sometimes warm to touch, and it's painful. All of these indicate your body is aware of the event and attempting to fix it. Now imagine that at the cellular level; at the microscopic level. The body recognizes an injury caused by some type of foreign body and the inflammatory response begins.

It is actually the presence of inflammation that makes most diseases symptomatic. Without the inflammation and the subsequent symptoms, a person wouldn't know about an illness or condition. The inflammatory response or process may persist for years before a person actually sees symptoms, and not all symptoms or conditions are auto-immune.

Many are conditions conventional medicine has a name for and a standard prescribed treatment. Arthr*itis*, diverticul*itis*, sinus*itis*, and so on. Notice the names of these conditions end with *"itis."* If you see these letters as a suffix, it tells you the disease is characterized by inflammation. So conventional doctors know the symptoms and they have a treatment. They don't always know the cause of the symptoms. Sometimes historically held beliefs and "concrete knowledge" come under fire. This is a challenge for many practitioners.

For my entire career I have worked with orthopedists (doctors who perform joint replace-ment surgeries and repair broken bones). I have met many I would say are excellent surgeons, and many are good friends. They spent long years and much money to become the surgeons who treat conditions like osteoarthritis (damage to the cartilage). If they are paying attention, they must now change their thinking. Consider the results of studies like the one published in the journal *Rheumatology* in 2011. Researchers now are learning the decades-long held belief that cartilage damage is the cause of osteoarthritis is not necessarily correct. What they have determined is the cause may be synov*itis*; inflammation of the synovial membrane that lines the joint.[45] They now have a different consideration when treating the pain, but they are still treating a symptom, in this case caused by inflammation.

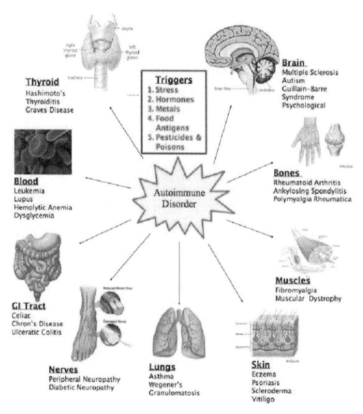

Figure 12 Illustration from www.TxFibro.com - a private online neuro-metabolic physician study group

There are many conditions researchers are still working to find the "cure" for. The research goes on and on, the money is spent, the drugs come to market, but people are just not getting well. We need to be treating the cause and *not* the symptoms.

I have included the graphic on the previous page to show some of the organs affected by inflammation and autoimmunity. As you can see, it includes virtually everything.

Those who have found answers and have overcome their symptoms and conditions are often anxious to share the approaches they took. The Internet is flush with personal stories on the part of medical practitioners, athletes, and mainstream individuals, from those with mild symptoms associated with food sensitivities all the way to people wheelchair bound and on disability due to the severity of their symptoms. Many sharing their stories have come to understand the cause of the problem, and want to share what they have done to correct the problem and their health. Interestingly, most of the stories have these things in common:

- Clean up the diet
- Identify and learn to avoid offending foods
- Make sure you detox
- Make sure you take lots of probiotics and digestive enzymes
- Reestablish healthy balance in the gut
- Take lots of good nutrients
- Get off the drugs

"Let food be thy medicine and medicine be thy food." That was Hippocrates over 2000 years ago. I think he was onto something.

CHAPTER 6

THE LARGE INTESTINE— A CLEAN COLON IS A HAPPY COLON

Once the chyme has traveled through the small intestine and most absorption of nutrients has taken place, the final breakdown products leave the small intestine and enter the large intestine where they are mixed with bacteria.

Anatomically, the large intestine is about five feet long, starting at the ileum and extending to the anus. At the ileum there is a fold of mucous membrane creating the *ileocecal valve* that regulates the passage of contents leaving the small intestine and entering the large intestine. The primary functions of the large intestine include:

- Completion of absorption
- Production of certain vitamins
- Formation of feces
- Expulsion of feces

Bacteria in the large intestine convert proteins into amino acids, break down the amino acids, and produce some B vitamins and vitamin K.

The four regions of the large intestine are the *cecum,* the *colon,* the *rectum,* and the *anal canal.* Below the ileocecal valve is the cecum. Attached to the cecum is a twisted, coiled tube measuring about three inches long called the *appendix,* or *vermiform appendix.* It contains lymphoid tissue and intercepts pathogenic (harmful) microorganisms that enter the digestive tract.

If fecal matter becomes trapped in the appendix, it may result in appendicitis (infection and inflammation), requiring an appendectomy to remove the inflamed appendix. The small end of the cecum merges with a long tube called the colon. The large intestine is often referred to as the colon. The colon comprises the largest part of the large intestine and is divided into the ascending colon, transverse colon, descending colon, and sigmoid portion (the left lower portion just before the rectum). The last eight inches make up the rectum which lies anterior (in front of) to the *sacrum* and *coccyx.* The final inch of the rectum is called the *anus.*

There are no villi or permanent circular folds in the mucosa of the large intestine. The epithelium or cell lining contains mostly absorptive and goblet cells. The goblet cells present on the inside lining secrete mucus. This mucus serves to lubricate the passage of contents through the colon.

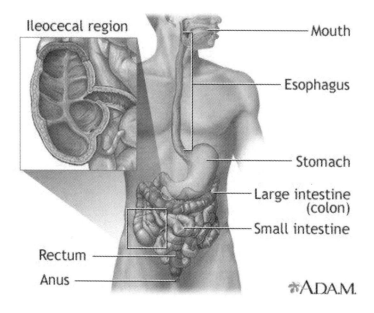

Ileocecal region

Mouth

Esophagus

Stomach

Large intestine (colon)

Small intestine

Rectum

Anus

*ADAM.

Figure 13 http://averaorg.adam.com/graphics/images/en/19293

The absorptive cells in the large intestine absorb mostly water. Ninety percent of water absorption occurs in the small intestine, leaving the final ten percent to be absorbed through the large intestine.

Although this is a relatively small amount, the large intestine is still an important organ for maintaining water and electrolyte balance. Anyone who has ever had diarrhea recognizes that losing so much water so quickly, along with all the electrolytes that are present, will dehydrate you and weaken you very quickly.

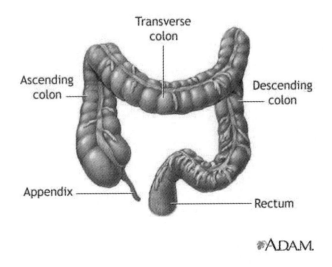

Figure 14 http://www.nlm.nih.gov/medlineplus/ency/images/ency/fullsize/8832

The large intestine also absorbs ions (atoms with a positive or negative charge) including sodium and chloride. Sodium has a positive charge and chloride has a negative charge. These help keep our electrolytes in balance. The large intestine also produces and absorbs some of the vitamins as noted above.

When seen by the naked eye the colon has a puckered appearance, the result of bands gathering into a series of pouches called *hostra*. Hostral churning accounts for the movement of chyme through the large intestine. As hostra become distended when they fill up, the walls contract and squeeze the contents into the next hostra. There is also peristaltic movement in the colon, but at a much slower rate than in the small intestine. Peristalsis in the large intestine averages 3 to 12 contractions per minute.

Mass peristalsis, a strong peristaltic wave, begins at about the middle of the transverse colon. This strong wave moves quickly to the rectum and the resulting distention of the rectal wall stimulates stretch receptors which initiate the defecation reflex that empties the rectum. Food in the stomach initiates this *gastrocolic* reflex in the colon, and if the digestive system is working properly, this mass peristalsis usually takes place during or immediately after each meal. Therefore, two to three bowel movements each day is optimal to keep the colon cleaned out. As babies, this happens automatically because voluntary control of the external annual sphincter has not yet developed.

Most people don't have two or three bowel movements a day. Many people would be very happy to have even one healthy bowel movement each day! Constipation and associated problems are on the rise. Many, including me, largely attribute this to our unhealthy diets, unhealthy eating habits, and unhealthy lifestyle.

As the chyme progresses through the large intestine, *Bifidobacterium* strains, residing primarily in the colon, digest substances in the chyme that are not digestible by the small intestines. Cellulose is a common constituent of a healthy diet, especially if raw vegetables are eaten. Human cells do not produce cellulase, the enzyme necessary to break down cellulose. However, several species of bacteria in the colon do synthesize cellulase, in turn digesting the cellulose. These bacteria lower the pH in the colon, keeping it an acidic environment and helping to protect and support the liver. In addition, they produce important vitamins including K, B1, B2, B6, B12, and biotin. Vitamin K is almost exclusively produced by gut bacteria and is essential for the proper clotting of blood. The end products of microbial digestion of cellulose and other carbohydrates are volatile fatty acids, lactic acid, methane, hydrogen, and carbon dioxide. This fermentation process is the major source of flatulence that leaves the body through the anus.

There are several chronic long-term health conditions that happen as a result of a poorly functioning lower digestive system. Crohn's disease, ulcerative colitis, irritable bowel syndrome, diverticulitis, and diverticulosis all are chronic long-term conditions starting in the gut.

One problem that is becoming more of an issue is chronic constipation. Many people suffer from chronic constipation and don't realize it, thanks to conventional medicine ignoring the necessity of a clean and healthy colon. I have worked taking care of patients for 40 years. Many times I overheard patients telling surgeons (after a colon surgery) that their normal routine was a bowel movement every two to three days. The surgeons would respond, if that is your routine that's fine and don't expect it will change. Every two to three days? Perhaps that's why they had to have colon surgery to begin with.

If all things are working properly, one should have at least two to three healthy bowel movements every day. I have worked with people who had a bowel movement once a week, sometimes once every ten days. What is happening when all that putrefied toxic waste is allowed to accumulate and stay in the colon? As blood circulates into the area to remove the final breakdown products of digestion, it circulates away full of toxins. Autointoxication develops and those toxins now have to be dealt with again by the immune system, the liver, and the kidneys.

Perhaps constipation, which is recognized as bowel movements that are infrequent or hard to pass, is a major problem. Functional medicine physicians feel each of us should have a bowel movement two to three times a day. What are some of the reasons we don't have frequent bowel movements?

Not Enough Water

Some believe water consumption to be highly overrated. After my years of experience caring for so many dehydrated and constipated patients, I recognize if we don't drink enough water, we become dehydrated *and* constipated. Some people tell me they get plenty to drink. However, much of what they drink is coffee, tea, and soda, all of which contribute to dehydration.

Water is necessary to maintain adequate blood pressure and circulating blood volume. It also moves toxins through the kidneys and colon. My general rule of thumb: take your total body weight in pounds, divide by two, and that is the number of ounces of water you should drink each day. Pure, filtered water with nothing added to it. If you are overweight, you should increase that by about 10 percent. If your job is heavy labor and you're perspiring all day, increase appropriately to maintain hydration and a general feeling of wellness. One common sign of dehydration is sluggishness. If you're sluggish, chances are you need a drink of water.

Not Enough Exercise

Now, I don't necessarily feel everyone needs to go join a gym and learn to pump iron. When I talk about exercise, I'm talking about some type of cardiovascular stimulation that will increase flow through the vascular system, which stimulates flow through the lymphatic system, thereby stimulating peristalsis through the gut. This can be simple cardio routines—stair stepping, walking, cycling—but, from my perspective, all within moderation. You should not find yourself having to walk 3 miles or stair-step for 50 minutes just to have a bowel movement.

Processed Foods

I am fond of saying "Stop eating the CRAP."

C – Caffeine and Carbonated beverages
R – Refined sugars and flours
A – Alcohol and Artificial sweeteners

P – Processed foods loaded with Preservatives

Some are appalled that I might use that acronym, but most people remember. When trying to maintain good overall health, and the health of your colon in particular, it is best to consider what you're putting into your body and best to consider eliminating these things.

Healthy Raw Foods

Eating lots of healthy fiber each day (this does not mean those popular, heavily advertised fiber products) will help move things through the colon in a more efficient manner.

The fibers I'm talking about are those that come from lots of healthy greens, vegetables, and fruits; not necessarily those coming from grains. Those five to eight servings a day of fresh fruits and vegetables are important for many reasons—including lots of vitamins and antioxidants—but providing healthy fiber is a big one.

Lack of Proper Elimination

What does this mean? Well, everyone is different, but as noted above if your gut is healthy you should expect two to three healthy bowel movements every day. Many people don't have those multiple healthy bowel movements daily. Part of the reason is because they don't take the time.

In their hurried world they get up, quickly take a shower, and choke down a cup of coffee, perhaps with artificial flavoring. If time permits, they perhaps heat up some toaster waffles, and head out the door, all without taking time to have a bowel movement. Then they go to work, perhaps in a public office building. Many people won't use a public toilet to have a bowel movement. There is some stigma associated with that, and I'm not exactly sure when it came to be. I question if it stems from a prim and proper Mother England as, after all, we sit on the throne to do our business.

So you don't have a bowel movement in the morning, and you don't have a bowel movement all day because of the environment you work in. Then you leave work, pick up the kids from basketball, baseball, ballet, or piano lessons, take them home, feed them the SAD diet, help them with their homework, put them to bed, and by the time it's time for you to sit down and relax, the urge is gone. The following day the vicious cycle repeats itself. All the while the putrefied toxic waste is accumulating and toxins are being recirculated. If this sounds familiar, reconsider what you are doing and come up with a way to take better care of you.

Another thing I discuss when talking about proper elimination is, again, the fact we sit on the throne. Having traveled to many different parts of the world, I'm fascinated by the approach other people take to this very normal, natural occurrence on the part of all humans. In some instances you'll walk up to the restroom facilities, the man will enter on the left, the woman enters on the right, and they meet in the middle.

I believe separate doorways are only to appease those of us who are used to going to the restroom that way. If meeting in the middle isn't shocking enough, you often find the little cleaning lady who's in there right with you. She continues to do her cleaning despite the fact you're in there to go to the bathroom. It doesn't matter to her, everyone does it.

One of the more fascinating experiences occurred when I was in Turkey. I love Turkey and can't wait to go back again someday. I walked up to the public restroom facility called a water closet. There was a big "WC" on the outside of the door, so I knew I was in the right place. However, when I opened the door, my first thought was where's the toilet? The toilet was, in fact, a hole in the ground with a very nice toilet seat covering the hole. To do your business, you squat over the hole and maintain that position.

Now if you don't have strong upper leg muscles, this could be a challenge. However, the interesting thing is anatomically, this is the healthiest position to assume while trying to evacuate the colon. The squatting position helps to relax the *puborectalis* muscle and straightens the rectum, rather than constricting it which is what happens when you sit.

Short of telling you to rip your toilets out of the floor, the recommendation I give most people is to purchase a stool that can be left in the bathroom. When it is time to have a bowel movement, sit on the commode, put your feet up on the stool so your knees are elevated above the level of your waist, and you will be assuming that proper anatomical position. There is at least one company I'm aware of that commercially produces these stools. This sophisticated stool can be purchased on the Internet.

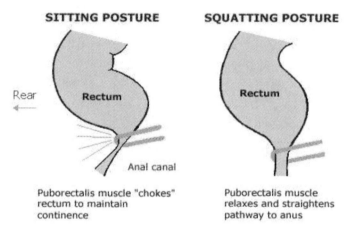

SITTING POSTURE   **SQUATTING POSTURE**

Rear

Rectum   Rectum

Anal canal

Puborectalis muscle "chokes" rectum to maintain continence

Puborectalis muscle relaxes and straightens pathway to anus

Figure 15 http://www.toilet-related-ailments.com/images/Puborectalis-Revised.jpg

Am I fond of colon cleansing? You bet! As I said in the beginning of this section, a clean colon is a happy colon. Our friend Hippocrates knew that over 2,000 years ago. He is credited with having said "Bad digestion is the root of all evil," and "Death begins in the colon."

When it comes to colon cleansing, there are many very good products on the market. I recommend a system that will not only help clean the putrefied toxic waste off the walls of the colon but will also help to kill parasites. Many people have parasites and don't know it. What we do know is parasites can contribute to a myriad of illnesses that can go undetected and undiagnosed for years.

I always enjoy taking the time to watch the TV show "The Monster Within Me." It is fascinating to learn what it ultimately takes to determine the diagnosis and course of treatment for the mysterious medical problems proven to result from parasites. I will be talking much more about parasites in my next book.

WHY IS AMERICA SO SICK?

PART II

CHAPTER 7

HORMONES—GUT HEALTH AND HORMONE FUNCTION

During Part I of this book, I discussed the role of a healthy gut and its relationship to a healthy immune system. Now, let me turn to a discussion of the role of a healthy gut and how it relates to a healthy hormonal system.

When we talk about the hormonal system, or the endocrine system as we know it, there is a lot to discuss. The entire system is very complex and regulates most of what happens in the body. By producing chemical messengers that circulate throughout the body, the endocrine system influences every organ and system. These chemical messengers are called hormones and are produced in the glands that make up the endocrine system. Hormones transfer information from one set of cells to another, depending on the job that needs to be done.

Let's start the discussion with hormones people are most familiar with, the sex hormones. All the symptoms associated with menopause have made this a very popular topic these days. Most of us have seen the TV commercials talking about those dreadful symptoms associated with menopause, and the latest new drug to treat the symptoms. For many women, listening is enough to convince you that you have a problem, and seeing your doctor to get that new drug is the best option, perhaps the only option.

Not so prevalent on TV is the popular topic of sex hormones relating to young people. More and more young couples are struggling to get pregnant. Currently in this country, for the most part there is at least one fertility clinic in every major city; some have many. When I was growing up, we didn't have fertility clinics and major studies. Having children was not a challenge for most, at least in the circles I ran in.

Today, fertility clinics are full of patients with major concerns related to the inability to conceive, or the inability to carry a healthy pregnancy to term if conception does occur. Researchers work tirelessly to determine if a gene is involved; or what needs to be done to increase the production of viable eggs in a female; or how to increase the production of healthy sperm in a male. People looking for the answers continue to deal in the same paradigm as researchers looking to create the next best pharmaceutical. They are treating the problem, but don't seem to consider the cause.

What is causing the problem? Much of it is our environment, the foods we eat that don't provide nutrition and are themselves part of the problem, the health of our gut, and the health of our immune system.

A Woman's Cycle

A woman's cycle begins on the first day of menses, the first day of bleeding. The first half of a woman's cycle is estrogen dominated and called the *follicular phase.* During the follicular phase of a woman's cycle, several *follicles* (fluid filled sacs in the ovaries) develop under the influence of FSH (follicle stimulating hormone). Each follicle contains an egg. In a typical cycle only one egg will become mature enough for ovulation. When a woman ovulates the egg will burst from the follicle. Then what is left of the follicle will become the corpus luteum. More estrogen is available, circulating and playing its role during that first half of the cycle.

Around day 12, the pituitary gland in the brain is responsible for secreting *luteinizing* hormone. Luteinizing hormone prepares and ripens the egg, getting it ready for release. During days 12 to 14 the ripening is taking place and, on approximately day 16, the egg is released. The *corpus luteum,* the temporary endocrine structure that forms when the egg is released from the follicle, begins to produce progesterone which starts to prepare the uterine lining, thickening it to make it ready for implantation of a fertilized egg. Adequate progesterone helps ensure a healthy pregnancy.

Women trying to get pregnant, or perhaps trying to get pregnant at a certain time, are encouraged to know when they ovulate. If the cycle is regular, a woman will start to check her temperature on day 14 to 16 to confirm ovulation is taking place. On about day 16, the egg is released and the corpus luteum begins to denature, causing a rise in progesterone and a concurrent rise in the basal body temperature. This indicates the egg has been released and is now traveling into and through the fallopian tubes and, ultimately, into the uterus to potentially be fertilized.

The remainder of the cycle, usually 28 to 32 days, is progesterone dominated and called the *luteal phase* (referring to the corpus luteum). The corpus luteum only lasts 12 to14 days, unless it gets the message a fetus is developing in the uterus. This message will come in the form of increasing HCG (human chorionic gonadotropin) from the developing fetus. If it gets the message it will continue to produce progesterone until the placenta takes over. If it does not receive that message, the corpus luteum dies and stops producing progesterone. As the progesterone level drops, the uterine wall stops thickening and begins to shed during menstruation.

There are other very important hormones that are helping to regulate this entire process. Around day 12, DHEA begins to rise as does testosterone. Some women don't realize that we have circulating testosterone, as it is mostly associated with men. However, starting after puberty, women produce adult levels of testosterone. This production is from both the ovaries and the adrenal glands, and is very important to help maintain muscle and bone mass.

It's interesting that testosterone begins to rise about day 12, considering that an appropriate level of testosterone is required to increase sex drive and, if we are actively attempting to procreate, sex drive is an important thing.

Before we go any further, an important consideration here is to recognize that these hormones are manufactured out of cholesterol. Without cholesterol, they cannot be produced in sufficient levels to regulate the bodily functions described. This would be one major reason you don't want to lower cholesterol. Think about it: estrogen, progesterone, testosterone, and DHEA are all called steroid hormones because they are produced from cholesterol. If you are not getting enough cholesterol in the diet, or you are artificially lowering your cholesterol taking a statin drug, what is the body to do? The body doesn't simply turn off its mechanism to create these hormones. It must get cholesterol somewhere.

The most readily available source of cholesterol in the human body is the *myelin sheath* of the brain, the covering that insulates the brain, spinal cord, and nerves that run throughout the body.

This is why many researchers concerned about the overuse of cholesterol-lowering drugs say there is a link between the use of these drugs, combined with prescribed low-fat/no-fat diets, and the rise in cases of Alzheimer's and dementia. If the body is going to pull cholesterol from the myelin sheath of the brain, that disrupts the functioning of the entire nervous system.

In addition, cholesterol comprises the cell membrane of every cell in the human body. During brain development, levels of cholesterol rise dramatically. Over the course of time they naturally decline. This implies that synthesis of cholesterol is necessary throughout life in order to maintain the healthy myelin sheath, and to allow nerves and nerve impulses to function properly. Lower cholesterol is a risk factor for certain neurodegenerative diseases.[46] Demyelination of the sheath, as the body robs it of cholesterol, leads to demyelination diseases like multiple sclerosis. As Dr. Joel D. Wallach points out in his book, *Epigenetics*, Alzheimer's disease is associated with the lowering of cholesterol. He cites the urgent FDA warning from April 2012 saying, "Statin drugs increase the risk of dementia and type 2 diabetes!"[47]

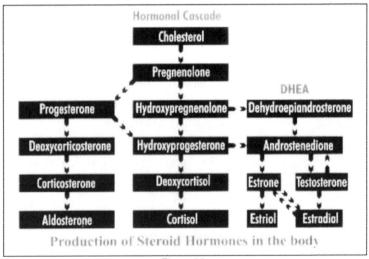

Figure 16
https://images.duckduckgo.com/iu/?u=http%3A%2F%2Fwww.natural-progesterone-advisory-network.com%2Fimages%2Fimage_pathway.jpg&f=1

Estrogen or estrogens? The human body actually produces three different types of estrogen as shown above. Estrone, estriol, estradiol.

The estradiol, or Beta 17 estradiol (E2 or 17β-estradiol), represents only about 10 percent of what the body produces. This form of estrogen drops to a very low but constant level after menopause. Beta 17 estradiol has the best binding site affinity, and therefore stays on the cell wall membrane for the longest period of time. Synthetic hormones are made with this particular estrogen.

Because it has the best binding site affinity, drug manufacturers elect to use this estrogen. However, staying longer on the cell wall membrane predisposes one to cancer. Drug manufacturers cannot patent drugs that are the actual hormone; it must be tweaked or altered in some way, so they create a synthetic form of the hormone as the drug. This form of Beta 17 estradiol is not the good, healthy estrogen.

Estriol is the healthy, beneficial estrogen. It constitutes approximately 80 percent of circulating estrogen. It is produced in large amounts by the placenta, the tissue that links the fetus to the mother, during pregnancy. It is a much safer estrogen with much lower binding site affinity, thereby staying on the cell wall membrane for a shorter period. As a result, it does not cause the problems with breast cancer that we see with Beta 17 estradiol. In fact, estriol is very protective against cancer of the breast and breast tissue.

Estrone is the third estrogen, making up approximately 10 percent of estrogen in the body. It is actually a "breakdown" hormone that dismantles estriol as well as Beta 17 estradiol, and is usually measured only during menopause and while testing for cancers of the testes, ovaries, or adrenals.

Women are wired to estrogen, whereas men are wired to testosterone. Healthy, circulating estrogens provide beneficial effects to the cardiovascular system (the heart and blood vessels). This is one reason why heart attack/heart failure rates rise after menopause, when we no longer have adequate amounts of circulating estrogen. Estrogen is also very protective of the brain and helps with improved cognitive function and memory. Estrogen also controls mood. One day we may be happy/sad, laughing/crying, or indifferent (we just don't care). Many women can relate to these emotions: being happy one minute and sad the next, laughing one minute and crying out of control for no reason five minutes later. Or we can feel totally indifferent; so it's suppertime and I forgot to take anything out of the freezer, oh well.

Estrogen is referred to as the anti-depressive hormone. If you have adequate amounts of circulating estrogen, you are likely to be one of those people who has a smile on and a bounce in your step. If your estrogen is low, chances are you are not that happy person, and no one would accuse you of having a bounce in your step.

The Second Half of a Woman's Cycle

This phase is progesterone dominated. As mentioned above, progesterone is released from the *corpus luteum* as it begins to deteriorate. Progesterone is also produced in the adrenal glands of both men and women. It is actually a major adrenal gland hormone. As noted, if the egg becomes fertilized, the corpus luteum will continue to produce progesterone until the placenta takes over.

Progesterone is responsible for several things, therefore we must have adequate progesterone as well as estrogen and testosterone. Progesterone stops the cellular growth of the uterus and is the hormone of pregnancy. If your progesterone level is not high enough, you may become pregnant, but not be able to hold the pregnancy. Progesterone is necessary for the implantation of the egg; even if the egg is fertilized, without adequate progesterone a woman cannot maintain a pregnancy. If the egg is not fertilized, progesterone begins to drop as the corpus luteum dies. The uterine lining stops thickening and is shed during menstruation.

Progesterone is also responsible for the secondary sex characteristics of a woman, and promotes the glandular development of the breast. As noted above, it increases the basal body temperature at the time of ovulation. It clears from the body very quickly.

One very important function of progesterone is it lowers estrogen's ability to bind with receptor sites. Therefore, it acts as a mild estrogen antagonist, helping to keep things in balance. The body must be in balance. Progesterone is considered the opposite of estrogen, therefore it is protective of what estrogen might cause. For example, estrogen primes the uterus, but progesterone is necessary to increase the uterine lining preparing for implantation of the egg. If the egg is not fertilized, the uterine lining sheds. The process ending either in fertilization of the egg and pregnancy, or not, requires hormones that are in balance. Progesterone is the antagonist of estrogen. Without adequate progesterone, as the antagonist, the uterine lining may continue to increase and ultimately cause uterine cancer.

Our bones go through a continual process of breakdown and rebuilding throughout our entire lives. The progesterone/estrogen balance is very important with respect to bone health. Estrogen promotes the cells called *osteoclasts*, which break down bone. Progesterone promotes the *osteoblasts*, the cells responsible for rebuilding bone.

To maintain a body in balance, other hormones are necessary as well. We have the *androgens* including testosterone and DHEA. In a woman, the ovaries secrete both. They are also produced in the adrenal glands. We mentioned earlier testosterone helps maintain muscle mass and helps increase sex drive. DHEA is often referred to as the "mother steroid" because it gives rise to all other hormones, both in the ovaries and the adrenals.

In the body we have different sources of hormones. We have the sex organs, which are the ovaries in women and the testes in men; the adrenal glands, responsible for producing these same hormones; and fat, which is also responsible for the production of estrogen, primarily Beta 17 estradiol. This is one reason there is much research on the link between obesity and breast cancer.[48]

The liver also plays a critical role in helping to keep everything in balance. Enzymes produced in the liver aid in the regulation of hormones while keeping things in balance, but only if the liver is healthy. We discussed earlier the effects of glyphosate (Roundup) on the CYP enzymes in the liver, and the potential hormonal disruption.[14] Several CYP enzymes are responsible for steroid hormone synthesis. All steroid hormones are produced from cholesterol by these same CYP enzymes.

Menopause

Menopause generally occurs in phases. First there is perimenopause, when a woman ovulates sometimes and not others, and has sporadic periods. Her periods may be erratic or incomplete, due to low progesterone levels that are not able to clear the uterine lining. Progesterone is sometimes referred to as the anti-witchy hormone because if there is plenty available, a woman is far less likely to have the mood swings so often associated with menopause. Hot flashes may start and symptoms may begin to seem or feel intolerable:

- Sleep disturbances

- Heart palpitations
- Dizziness
- Memory loss
- Vaginal dryness/painful intercourse
- Changes in glucose tolerance
- Decreased sex drive
- Changes in body shape (the body is trying to put on fat to produce more estrogen)
- Coronary artery disease
- Abnormal uterine bleeding
- Migraine headaches
- Hot flashes
- Mood changes

These can make for a very miserable time in a woman's life.

Menopause is recognized and diagnosed when a woman has not had menses for one year. Menopause should be a very normal, natural event. If everything is in balance, if the system is working properly, and if the adrenals are not fatigued, a women may well go through menopause without any symptoms. In today's world that is rarely the case.

We generally see women running off to their physician or OB/GYN, and the recommendation is often hormone replacement therapy. You're not likely to find a conventional OB/GYN who's going to tell you to clean up your diet and repair your gut. However, hormone replacement therapy has become controversial. Due to problems with cancers related to synthetic hormone replacement therapy, many docs choose not to recommend that form of therapy. Some, however, still prescribe synthetic hormone replacement therapy,[49] a practice felt by many to be very risky.

Synthetic hormone replacement therapy is Prempro, Provera, or Premarin, and comes in the form of pills, skin patches, ointments, injections, etc. Interestingly enough, these synthetic hormone replacement drugs are made using pregnant mares' urine, thus the names. The structure of the estrogen is not exactly the same as the human form, and these drugs do not use progesterone; 3-methyl progesterone is used instead. Many side effects occur because these synthetic hormones do not bind efficiently and effectively to the cell wall. These drugs come with a concerning list of side effects and are prescribed by most physicians with the "benefits outweigh the risks philosophy." After all, what is a girl to do? She can't be expected to add the stressful symptoms of the "change" to all the other stress in her life.

Male Menopause

Now if you're a man reading this, your time has come. Men experience what we call male menopause, correctly named *andropause.* This time in a man's life is often referred to as "midlife crisis." It is a transitional period for men when they experience what is termed the "second childhood." Some men do well with this phase of their lives; others have to go find a fast car, or perhaps a fast woman, to help them deal with the changes they are experiencing. These events usually begin around age 40 to 45, followed by rapid deterioration of symptoms after age 50.[50] The phase is called andropause because the symptoms coincide with the decrease in the class of male hormones called the androgens.

The hallmark of andropause is decreasing testosterone levels when measured in the blood. Symptoms accompany several physiological changes that are commonly associated with aging. These changes include:

- Diminished libido
- Decreased frequency of sex ("senior slump")
- Erectile dysfunction
- Infertility
- Changes in body composition
- Reduction in body and facial hair and
- Osteoporosis

Andropause is, in effect, the reverse of puberty.

Men report increasing levels of anger, confusion, depression, and fatigue that are significantly higher than those reported by men with normal testosterone levels.

For a long time, andropause was not recognized by conventional medicine. Many middle-aged men have shared with me their suffering of these symptoms. Because they were concerned, they would visit their physicians, only to be told it was probably stress. Many were given an antidepressant, and/or perhaps a sleeping pill. Those drugs would only serve to mask the symptoms, never really dealing with the underlying problems.

Just as with women, men should go through this phase in their lives normally and naturally. So often, that is not the case, and men feel their only hope is to get those "drugs." There are plenty of them out there to help deal with the issues and stresses associated with andropause. If erectile dysfunction is an issue, just watch TV around the time of the six o'clock news and you will learn of several choices. I caution you to not have the kids in the room, because answering that question about an erection lasting longer than four hours can sometimes be awkward.

Now if you just don't have the drive, there are testosterone replacements. You may have the choice of a pill or, perhaps, a "roll-on" like deodorant. Caution, there are more and more commercials now directing you to legal assistance if you have suffered any of the serious side effects associated with some of these drugs.

It is important to understand these problems are common, but they do not result from a deficiency of Viagra, just like heart disease is not a deficiency of Lipitor or Crestor (although you might think so if you watch too many commercials). Many of these problems are because you are getting older, and hormone levels do drop as one ages.

In the body, we have mechanisms and systems that are designed to support and regulate these changes. If those mechanisms function normally, a person may not realize they have gone through the change.

The Adrenal Glands

The primary support system in the body when it comes to hormones is the adrenal glands. They are a very important part of the endocrine system. Again, the endocrine system is the system made up of all the glands responsible for the release of all the messengers called hormones. Below is a diagram showing the glands that make up the endocrine system.

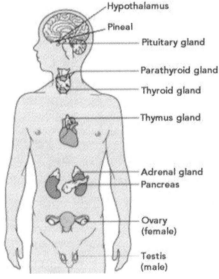

Figure 17 http://www.endoatsoim.com/images/endocrine_system.jpg

See how all this works in concert, if you will. The hypothalamus releases the hormone cortico-trophin-releasing hormone (CRH), which stimulates the pituitary gland to release adrenal corticotrophin hormone (ACTH), which in turn stimulates the adrenal glands to produce corticosteroid hormones.

The adrenal glands, as you see in the diagram, are two very small glands that sit on top of the kidneys. Each is made up of two distinct parts. The adrenal cortex is the outside or the outer part of the gland, and it produces hormones considered vital to life. One is *cortisol* which helps regulate metabolism, helps the body respond to stress, and regulates how the body converts fats, proteins and carbohydrates to energy. *Corticosteroid* hormones are also pro-duced. Along with *hydrocortisone* (cortisol), these regulate the immune system response and suppress inflammatory reactions. These hormones are called *glucocorticoid* hormones.

The adrenal cortex also releases the primary *mineralocorticoid* hormone known as aldosterone, responsible for maintaining water and salt balance along with healthy blood pressure. The adrenal cortex is also responsible for releasing the sex steroids (sex hormones) in small amounts in healthy young adults. During youth, the ovaries and testes produce the majority of these. As we age, if the adrenals are working well, and are not overworked and fatigued, they take over the job.

The inner part of the adrenal gland is called the *adrenal medulla* and it produces non-essential hor-mones (those that are not necessary for you to live).

These are released after the sympathetic nervous system is stimulated. The most familiar is probably *epinephrine,* also called *adrenaline,* which prepares your body to spring into action during a stressful situation. This is known as the "fight or flight" response, a process initiated by the sympathetic nervous system when the body encounters a stressful or threatening situation. When adrenaline is released there is an increase in heart rate and a rushing of blood to the muscles and to the brain. This also causes a spike in blood sugar by helping convert glycogen to glucose in the liver.

Norepinephrine, or *noradrenaline,* is the other hormone in the medulla and it works with epinephrine in response to stress. Noradrenaline is responsible for vasoconstriction (narrowing of the blood vessels). In turn, this elevates blood pressure. In this way, your body can effectively deal with stress. Problems arise, however, with the function of the adrenal glands when they must constantly respond to stress, either high-level stress period-ically, or low-level stress on a continual basis. When this happens, the adrenal glands become fatigued.

The adrenal glands are also responsible for keeping minerals in balance; controlling absorption through the membrane of the gut; regulating blood sugar levels by controlling the release of glucose and stored glycogen in the liver; and producing DHEA, the mother hormone giving rise to the other hormones. If the adrenal glands are fatigued these critical functions do not occur effectively. You may develop symptoms of fatigue, mood changes, digestive problems, and the inability to handle stress of any kind, physical or emotional. You may have a decreased sex drive; you may gain or lose weight.

Chances are if you go to the doctor with any of these symptoms, you are likely to have a workup done which will include blood work. However, the adrenals are not often suspected as the cause of the problem. Caring for patients in the hospital for many years, adrenal fatigue was not suggested or addressed as a diagnosis or concern unless the person had a diagnosed adrenal condition such as Addison's disease, Cushing's syndrome, adrenal cancer, etc. Recent research has brought adrenal fatigue to the forefront in functional medicine, and all-natural treatments for adrenal fatigue are yielding impressive results. Some effective all-natural treatments include cleaning up the diet and getting rid of the hormone disrupters. GM foods must be eliminated to curtail the damage done to the CYP enzymes that are responsible for steroid hormone synthesis. As mentioned previously, these vital hormones are produced from cholesterol by CYP enzymes.

So, the adrenal glands in their role as the stress glands have a major job trying to keep us in balance, in addition to the responsibility of producing all the sex hormones and other hormones. In response to our everyday stress, the adrenal glands are busy balancing all the reactions, as well as keeping us regulated by communicating with the other glands and all other organ systems throughout the body. All of this work may lead to adrenal fatigue. The stress caused by hormonal imbalance during perimenopause and menopause can be a huge factor in adrenal fatigue. Is it any wonder menopausal women are often said to have a short fuse?

Thyroid Function

Although the endocrine glands are all-important, each with their critical role to play, there are certain relationships among the glands that deserve special mention. As discussed, the adrenal glands produce many hormones; DHEA, estrogen, hydrocortisone, progesterone, pregnanolone and testosterone. Each of these hormones interacts with thyroid hormone in the body.

Our thyroid gland, responsible for our metabolic rate, produces two major hormones: *thyroxine* (T4) and *triiodothyronine* (T3). This production occurs when the pituitary gland produces a hormone called thyroid stimulating hormone, or TSH, which in turn stimulates the thyroid gland to produce these hormones. The thyroid gland produces much more T4 than T3, but T3 is much more active than T4. Iodine is required for the thyroid to produce these hormones and, in fact, the T4 has four iodine molecules attached to it and the T3 has three iodine molecules.

T3 is the hormone that actually increases the metabolism inside the cells. The majority of T4 is actually converted into T3 inside the cells of the body. When the body has adequate amounts of thyroid hormone available, TSH levels are lowered so the thyroid gland can lower its production of the hormones.

This is all monitored through a series of lab tests. Unfortunately, the way testing is done in most situations is incomplete. Oftentimes what is checked is a person's TSH. If the TSH is elevated, this indicates the pituitary gland is sensing low thyroid hormone levels in the body. TSH is being secreted in order to stimulate the thyroid gland to produce more thyroid hormone.

If the TSH is normal, however, many physicians believe that automatically rules out a hypothyroid state. Patients are told they are not hypothyroid, despite the fact they may have many of the symptoms associated with hypothyroidism. Some common symptoms include:

- Weight gain
- Dry skin and brittle nails
- Hair loss
- Fatigue
- Menstrual irregularities and infertility
- Puffy eyes and eyelids
- Irritability and inability to concentrate

To have some or all of these symptoms and be told you have a normal thyroid can be frustrating.

It is more accurate to check the free T3 and T4 levels as well. T3 is the active thyroid hormone that gets into the cells to maintain metabolism. The TSH is more reflective of T4 levels, which is often a poor indicator of true thyroid function.

As mentioned, T4 must be converted to T3. However, in many individuals the T3 is suppressed. So unless we determine exactly what the T4 and T3 are, many people who have hypothyroid may go undiagnosed. If hypothyroid is diagnosed, standard protocol is to continue to monitor lab work and continue to prescribe medication based on what the lab is showing.

This leads to several problems down the line, as many people who are treated with thyroid medication are given a synthetic form such as Levothyroxine. Synthetic forms of a medication do not function the same way in the human body as a natural form of the medication would. Many people who are truly hypothyroid can never get adequately regulated and never feel healthy a day in their lives. I am of the opinion that the natural form of thyroid is necessary, such as Armor thyroid. Many physicians are unfamiliar with what it takes to regulate a person on a natural thyroid medication. It is much easier for them to just prescribe the synthetic form and adjust the dose according to the lab work. Again without any discussion concerning cleaning up the diet or improving gut function both of which have shown great promise for patients with both hypo- or hyperthyroid issues.

Let's consider that perhaps there's not enough thyroid hormone. What happens when the adrenal messengers attempt to send signals to thyroid messengers? If the adrenals are stressed there is an inadequate production of adrenal hormone. This can result in poor conversion of the active thyroid hormone T4 into the more active thyroid hormone T3.

By the same token, when thyroid hormone is prescribed for a hypothyroid condition, metabolism is increased. This increased metabolism will, in turn, stimulate the adrenal glands to secrete the hormone hydrocortisone or cortisol. Cortisol is necessary to mobilize glucose out of the cells in order to supply energy to each cell in the body. If the adrenal glands are not able to increase the production of adrenal hormone because of a hypo-adrenal state or adrenal exhaustion, increasing the metabolism with thyroid hormone will in turn overload the poorly functioning adrenal gland and precipitate a failure of the adrenal glands. The ultimate consequence of this failure can be severe; adrenal failure is incompatible with life.

Further, there is the consideration of thyroid function and specific compounds responsible for disrupting thyroid hormones. These would include the common hormone disruptors:

- Bisphenol-A (BPA)
- PCBs
- Triclosan (look at your anti-bacterial hand soap and dish detergent)
- Phthalates
- Fire retardants
- Pesticides
- Synthetic hormones
- Artificial sweeteners

These all are common sources of endocrine disruption.[51] These are many of the things we are exposed to every day if we consume the SAD diet, ensure the house smells like a spring meadow, kill all the bacteria we can (good and bad) while increasing the overgrowth and mutation of all bacteria, eat canned foods, and use plastic containers and so on.

In my opinion, the genesis of "Better Living Through Chemistry" has often harmed more than helped the human race. Some would argue there have been vast improvements as a result of the lab experiments and creations on the part of chemical company giants like Monsanto, Dow and DuPont. Just look at all the new cleaning supplies, flame retardants, air fresheners, plastic food storage containers, laundry care products and other conveniences created with reckless abandon and no consideration for potential side effects of the chemicals used in their making.

I think we have been shown time and time again, products are rushed to market and it is only after a few years of exposure, sometimes not that long, we start to struggle with concerns. That's not important to companies if there is money to be made. These chemical *wonders* are presented to us under the guise of making our world a better place; making life good, better, or the best it can be. Many changes resulting from creating a more convenient world, are killing us. When I did radio I was fond of saying, "If God or Mother Nature made it, it is good but if man made it, it is questionable at best."

The studies are out there and the facts make it so. These hormone disruptors mimic our hormones and cause profound changes resulting in everything from obesity, cardiovascular disease, liver disease, pancreatitis, neurological diseases, and the other conditions mentioned here and many not mentioned. Giving our endocrine system all these extra hormone mimicking chemicals throws the entire, interconnected system out of balance affecting all other systems in the body. To be healthy, everything must be in balance.

CONCLUSION

Writing this book has been a source of joy for me. It has given me the opportunity to put on paper many of the things I like to share with people. I believe knowledge is power and many times because we don't know, what we don't know, we lack the power to effect positive changes in our health.

I approach all-natural medicine from a very unique perspective. Having worked in the medical field for 40 years, I had the opportunity to experience Western medicine/conventional medicine working in the trenches, if you will. My knowledge does not come from some articles I read. I was there. I saw it happen. I had the experience and I can share those experiences.

The message I hope to convey is: *you are in control*. Western medicine is important and certainly plays a critical role when it comes to trauma and emergency situations. Heaven knows I was very thankful for highly skilled and trained Western medical docs right there with me in the emergency room and right there with me while caring for and transporting brave men and women injured on the battlefield.

My disquiet is with so many chronically sick people who say, "My doctor knows best" or "I'll do whatever my doctor says, he's/she's been so won-derful to me."

From my all-natural perspective I don't feel that is the best approach to personal health care. Yet, many people feel this way. "The doctors treating me know a lot more about the body than I do." That may be true but they don't know everything about *your* body.

Many people are compelled to feel, "my doctor knows best" because of the way they are treated by their doctors. I've watched MDs tell patients, "if you don't want to do what I've suggested you can find yourself another doctor" or, "this is the best I have to offer, take it or leave it, I'm the doctor here, and I know better than you." When you are sick and afraid and you don't know why, these words can be very harsh and make you feel much worse.

You are in control! It is your body and your life and you should be able to make decisions about the proper maintenance and care of the body you will spend your life in. You need to be able to make informed decisions and that is why I've written this book. I realize that many of the problems people have, they have because they just don't know. There's a saying I will often use that goes like this, "I'm sorry people feel that way, they don't know what they don't know."

Conventional medicine does not always have the answer and does not always know what's best. If they did, we wouldn't have so many chronically ill patients making repeat visits to their physicians for repeat prescription refills. Conventional medicine is treating the symptoms, not treating the cause. In so many cases the symptoms are not difficult to understand if you know the cause. Further, understanding more about the simple steps you can take to avoid the cause can lead you down a path of health and wellness.

Often times, it's the simple things like understanding what's in your food or the medications you're taking. Most are harmful; not healthful but if you are not aware of that, you will continue to expose yourself, your family and loved ones to the harmful things that create chronic illness. There was a study released a few years ago in *The New England Journal of Medicine*, a prestigious medical journal that told us this is the first generation whose parents will outlive their children.[52] How sad is that?

We need to start educating the consumer and start putting them on the road to wellness.

I work with clients every day and my approach is relatively simple.

Clean up the diet. Remove the things found to be harmful: gluten, GMOs, excessive caffeine, carbonated beverages, refined sugars and flours, alcohol, and processed foods loaded with preservatives. Eat clean, organic, whole foods.

Cleanse from different perspectives (colon, liver, kidneys, tissues and organs). Cleaning out what has contributed to ill health is a great way to start.

Reestablish good healthy gut function. After cleansing take plenty of quality digestive enzymes and probiotics to flood the system with those beneficial bacteria and assist with optimal digestion. You are what you digest.

Ensure you are taking what I consider to be the 90 essential nutrients every organ, cell, and tissue in the body require. Not all supplements are created equal; taking quality supplements is most beneficial. Taking lesser quality supplements is harmful.

Drink plenty of good clean, filtered water.

Get plenty of sleep. Learn to take time for yourself and learn to be quiet and meditate.

This may seem like a lot but I encourage you to start somewhere. Even the small changes will be of benefit and as health improves, the bigger changes come more easily for most.

It is often a challenge to put the pieces together and determine a program that will work best for you. I have worked with many clients who are struggling because they are so sick and can't find the answers. They are desperate to feel better and many have spent much time and money finding the right doctor, having all the tests to find what might work and spending more money on supplements offered based on lab results seeing no results.

My approach is different. Knowing lab results that fall outside the normal range indicated the body has done everything it can to correct and maintain, encourages me to take a simpler approach. For example, if your serum calcium level is determined to be low that means your body has done all it can to help maintain that normal level.   You would most likely be told you need to supplement with calcium. That sounds simple enough but you need the right type of calcium and the proper amount of magnesium and the other co-factors to make that calcium work and to keep everything in balance. If you decide to just take a calcium supplement, you may well put other things out of balance. Just taking calcium is not helpful and may be dangerous.

The body must always be in balance. Given that, my approach is to start with recognizing the foods that may be problematic to thereby adjust toward a more healthy diet. As I said, I feel cleansing is important and depending on the person and symptoms, I will recommend various cleanses to achieve the desired results. I follow with a healthy gut restoration program while supplementing with all known nutrients. Whole food source vitamins, minerals and trace minerals in a colloidal form, and so forth, so the supplements are easily absorbed and readily available to be used by the body. I have developed symptom specific protocols based on my experiences working with hundreds of people who have themselves determined conventional medicine is not their best choice, because it is not working.

As I said earlier, knowledge is power and understanding how and why an all-natural approach helps maintain balance and why improvements are seen using this approach, and not the pharmaceutical and surgical approach, has led to many regaining their vitality and health in a very short period of time.

In addition to the basics, my recommendations may also include herbs and essential oils as I feel there are several ways to effect a change and supporting all systems by various means will help create and maintain a body in balance. For more information and to learn more about my protocols and recommendations visit www.drjconaway.com.

I have seen amazing differences, amazing changes in the health and wellness of so many people. I recommend natural therapies to promote optimal health and am proud to conclude that with sound knowledge and positive steps, people can enjoy life; feeling vibrant and healthy well into their later years. You don't have to fear getting older because you don't have to fear the consequences of being sick.

TO YOUR BEST HEALTH!

INDEX

beta 17 estradiol, 133-134, 137

bifidobacterium, 87, 115

bile, 60, 72, 76-80, 82-83, 86

C

caffeine, 93, 96, 118, 155

calcium, 50, 52-54, 156-157

candida, 90-92, 97

carbohydrate, 3, 27, 46, 58, 62-63, 71-72, 78, 143

CCK, 60, 74, 82

celiac disease, 15, 26

cholecystokinin, 60, 74, 82

cholesterol, 76-82, 86, 91, 131-132, 137, 145

chyme, 55, 57, 69-73, 111, 114-115

colon, 90, 111-112, 114-117, 119, 121, 122, 155

corn, 28-31, 35-36, 46, 96

cortisol, 81, 143, 149

CYP, 78-82, 134, 145

cytochrome P450, 78-79

D

DHEA, 81, 130-131, 136, 144, 146

digestion, 43-45, 47, 52, 54-56, 58, 60, 64, 67-73, 82-83, 87, 97, 116-117, 122, 156

digestive enzymes, 50, 54, 62, 66-67, 73-74, 101, 108, 155

dysbiosis, 92, 97

glycogen, 78, 144

glyphosate, 29-30, 32, 78-79, 81-80, 137

GM, 28-31, 35, 78-79, 82, 145

GMO, 28, 31-33, 35-36, 46, 78, 80, 96, 155

gut, 26, 30, 79, 87-95, 98, 100-102, 104-105, 108, 116, 118-119, 127, 129, 138, 144, 148, 155, 157

gut flora, 87, 89

gut microbiome, 88, 94-93

gut microbiota, 87, 89

H

HCl, 51-52, 57, 59-60, 67

hormonal, 81, 91, 127, 137, 146

hormone, 34, 47, 54, 56, 60, 73-74, 78, 81-82, 94, 127-131, 133-149, 151

hormone replacement therapy, 138-139

human genome, 18-19, 88

hyperthyroid, 148

hypothyroid, 147-149

I

immune system, 67, 92, 94, 96, 98-99, 101-103, 105, 117, 127, 129, 143

inflammation, 30, 90, 94, 106-108, 112

inflammatory, 105-106, 143

L

lactic acid, 116

pepsin, 45, 56, 60-61, 65

peristalsis, 49, 55, 91-92, 114-115, 118

permeable, 26, 103, 105

pregnanolone, 146

probiotics, 4, 87-88, 96, 100-101, 108, 155

progesterone, 129-132, 135-137, 139, 146

prostaglandins, 94

protein, 3, 17-18, 22, 25-27, 29-30, 37, 52-53, 56, 58, 60-63, 65, 71-72, 78, 80, 91, 102, 112, 143

R

Roundup, 29, 79-80, 137

S

SAD, 41-43, 46, 68, 78, 93, 96, 120, 150

soy, 27, 29-31

Standard American Diet, 41, 46, 93

steroid hormones, 81, 131, 137

steroids, 34, 79, 81, 92, 96, 99, 143

stomach, 44-47, 49-61, 65-66, 69-70, 73, 75, 93, 96, 115

stress, 67, 74, 93-95, 104, 139-140, 143-146

stress glands, 145

T

T3, 146-149

T4, 144-149

T cells, 102-103

About the Author

Joanne M. Conaway, N.D. has a unique perspective of medicine and healthcare, having started her career as a nurse earning her Bachelor of Science Degree in Nursing in 1976. Her experiences span all medical disciplines, having started in the ER and continuing in Operating Room, Critical Care, Cardiac Care, and Nutritional Support. These experiences afforded her the opportunity to observe the human body from various aspects health and disease. While doing Nutritional Support, she cared for people who could no longer eat by mouth, receiving all their nutrition intravenously or by tube feeding. Dr. Conaway gained an in-depth understanding of nutrition at the cellular level and the importance of gastrointestinal system function. This understanding and experience sparked her passion for helping people understand the importance of a healthy diet and a healthy gastrointestinal system.

Dr. Conaway is a retired Lieutenant Colonel. She spent 20 years in the U.S. Air Force and Air Force Reserves, primarily as an Aeromedical Evacuation Nurse in Training/Standardization, while serving as in-flight Medical Crew Director. During her career, she deployed in support of "Operation Just Cause" in Panama and "Operation

Desert Storm" in the European Theater in support of a major staging facility.

As an internationally acclaimed speaker and author, some of her most popular lectures are *"You Are What You Digest," "Inches of Deception,"* and *"Why Is America So Sick? Understanding the Gastrointestinal / Hormone Link."* She has coordinated, developed, and taught nutrition education courses for professional organizations and corporations as well as Continuing Medical Education courses for medical professionals. Her primary focus is the function of the gastrointestinal system, its role in overall health, and how it specifically relates to immunity, autoimmunity, and hormonal issues in both men and women.

With over 40 years in the health care industry, Dr. Conaway has learned that although it often seems the scientific world is making strides toward "cures" in many areas such as cancer and heart disease, there is more to health and wellness. Diseases are not a deficiency of prescription drugs and over-the-counter medications. Dr. Conaway is convinced that humans are not created to begin deteriorating at 40 or 50; growing older does not automatically lead to medical problems. She has learned that so much of what adversely impacts our health and wellness is our environment and lifestyle; primarily our food supply. Her opinion is based on her experiences and her understanding of nutritional needs and the lack of healthy nutritionals in our diets.

Dr. Conaway was no longer willing to do the work expected of her in mainstream medicine because of conflicts between the conventional approach of treating symptoms with pharmaceuticals and what she feels is a better approach, that is, preventing and healing using all-natural means such as nutritional supplements, herbal formulas, and essential oils. She has retired from traditional medicine, consults privately, and for 16-plus years has worked with a nutrition company, currently serving on its Scientific Advisory Board. Dr. Conaway believes very strongly as humans we are body, mind, and spirit, and her approach addresses each of these on a path to wellness. She is frequently invited to share her views as a guest and guest host on popular radio shows.

Dr. Conaway currently lives in upstate New York with her husband Rich and their son, Rhett. She is available for lectures, radio, television interviews, and private consultations, sharing her message of health.

REFERENCES

[1] Preamble to the Constitution of the World Health Organization as adopted by the International Health Conference, New York, 19-22 June, 1946; signed on 22 July 1946 by the representatives of 61 States (Official Records of the World Health Organization, no. 2, p. 100) and entered into force on 7 April 1948.

[2] http://www.cdc.gov/media/releases/2014/p0327-autism-spectrum-disorder.html

[3] http://www.cdc.gov/ncbddd/adhd/data.html

[4] http://www.cdc.gov/diabetes/statistics/prev/national/figage.htm

[5] http://www.mayo.edu/research/discoverys-edge/celiac-disease-rise

[6] http://www.alz.org/alzheimers_disease_facts_and_figures.asp#quickFacts

[7] *National Human Genome Research Institute (NHGRI) http://www.genome.gov/*

[8] https://medium.com/the-physics-arxiv-blog/human-genome-shrinks-to-only-19-000-genes-21e2d4d5017e

⁹ Lipton, Bruce H., *The Biology of Belief: Unleashing the Power of Consciousness, Matter and Miracles*, Mountain of Love Productions, Inc. and Elite Books, San Rafael, CA 2005

¹⁰ http://www.theguardian.com/commentisfree/2011 /apr/17/human-genome-genetics-twin-studies

¹¹ Davis, William, M.D., *"Wheat Belly – Lose The Wheat, Lose The Weight and Find Your Path Back to Health,"* Rodale, New York 2011

¹² Perlmutter, David, M.D. and Loberg, Kristin, *"Grain Brain: The Surprising Truth about Wheat, Carbs, and Sugar-- Your Brain's Silent Killers,"* Little Brown and Company Hachette Book Group, New York 2013

¹³ http://gmo-awareness.com/all-about-gmos/gmo-defined/

¹⁴ http://gmo-awareness.com/all-about-gmos/gmo-defined/

¹⁵ National Agricultural Statistics Board annual report, 30 June 2010. Retrieved 23 July 2010. http://usda.mannlib.cornell.edu/usda/nass/Acre/2010 s/2010/Acre-06-30-2010.pdf

¹⁶ Samsel, Anthony and Seneff, Stephanie, *Glyphosate's Suppression of Cytochrome P450 Enzymes and Amino Acid Biosynthesis by the Gut Microbiome: Pathways to Modern Diseases*, Entropy, 18 April 2013

¹⁷ http://www.fda.gov/aboutfda/whatwedo/

[18] Drucker, Steven M., *Altered Genes, Twisted Truth: How the Venture to Genetically Engineer Our Food Has Subverted Science, Corrupted Government, and Systematically Deceived the Public*, Clear River Press, Salt Lake City, UT, 2015

[19] Laufer, Peter *"Organic: A Journalist's Quest to Discover the Truth behind Food Labeling"* Globe Pequot Press, Guilford, CT, 2014

[20] http://www.consumerreports.org/cro/2014/10/where-gmos-hide-in-your-food/index.htm

[21] http://www.yourhormones.info/hormones/ghrelin.aspx

[22] Logemann JA., *Evaluation and Treatment of Swallowing Disorders*, 2nd ed. PRO-ED Austin, TX 1998

[23] H. S. Callahan, D. E. Cummings, M. S. Pepe, P. A. Breen, C. C. Matthys, and D. S. Weigle, *Postprandial suppression of plasma ghrelin level is proportional to ingested caloric load but does not predict intermeal interval in humans,* Journal of Clinical Endocrinology and Metabolism, vol. 89, no. 3, pp. 1319–1324, 2004.

[24] http://www.elmhurst.edu/~chm/vchembook/571lockkey.html

[25] http://www.vivo.colostate.edu/hbooks/pathphys/digestion/smallgut/anatomy.html

[26] Loomis, Howard F., **Jr.,** *Enzymes: The Key to Health, Vol. 1 The Fundamentals,* Paperback – August, 2005, 21st Century Nutrition Publishing, Madison Wisconsin, 2007

[27] Howell, Dr. Edward, *Enzyme Nutrition: The Food Enzyme Concept - Unlocking the Secrets for Eating Right for Health, Vitality and Longevity* Avery, 1985

[28] http://www.vivo.colostate.edu/hbooks pathphys/digestion/liver/bile.htm

[29] http://people.cornellcollege.edu/bnowakthompson /pdfs/liverDetox.pdf

[30] Nebert, D.W., Russell, D.W. *Clinical importance of the cytochromes P450. The Lancet* 2002, *360*, 1155–1162.

[31] Wikvall, K. *Cytochrome P450 enzymes in the bioactivation of vitamin D to its hormonal form* (review). *Int. J. Mol. Med.* 2001, *7*, 201–209.

[32] Richard, S.; Moslemi, S.; Sipahutar, H.; Benachour, N.; S'eralini, G.E., Differential effects of glyphosate and Roundup® on human placental cells and aromatase. *Environ. Health Perspect.* 2005, *113*, 716–720.

[33] http://academy.asm.org/images/stories/documents /FAQ_Human_Microbiome.pdf

[34] Pappas, Stephanie, *Your Body Is a habitat ... for Bacteria.* Science Now Daily News, 2009

[35] Berg, R,. *"The indigenous gastrointestinal microflora".* Trends in Microbiology 4, 1996

[36] Hecht G., Innate mechanisms of epithelial host defense: spotlight on intestine. *Am. J. Physiol. Cell Physiol.*277(3),C351–C358 1999

[37] http://www.globalhealingcenter.com/natural-health/chlorine-cancer-and-heart-disease

[38] Koontz D, Hinze, J et al 1999, "Leaky Gut Syndrome", Origins, Effects and Therapies, The Medical Link Between Dysbiosis and Many Major Ailments' The Herbal Pharm 19, pp 8

[39] Bjarnason I, Macpherson AJ, 1994, "NSAIDs cause small intestinal inflammation in 65% of patients receiving the drugs long-term." Intestinal toxicity of non-steroidal anti-inflammatory drugs. Pharmacology Therapy Apr-May;62(1-2) pp145-57

[40] http://www.apa.org/monitor/2012/09/gut-feeling.aspx

[41] http://www.rodalenews.com/gut-health

[42] Dumas ME, Maibaum EC, Teague C *et al*, Assessment of analytical reproducibility of 1H NMR spectroscopy based metabonomics for large-scale epidemiological research: the INTERMAP Study. *Anal. Chem.*78(7),2199–2208, 2006

[43] Bailey MT, Dowd SE, Galley JD, Hufnagle AR, Allen RG, Lyte M., Exposure to a social stressor alters the structure of the intestinal microbiota: Implications for stressor-induced immunomodulation. *Brain Behav. Immun.*25(3),397–407, 2011

[44] http://www.niaid.nih.gov/topics/immuneSystem/immuneCells/Pages/tcells.aspx

[45] Sofat N[1], Ejindu V, Kiely P., *What Makes Osteoarthritis Painful? The Evidence for Local and Central Pain Processing*, Rheumatology (Oxford) 2011 Dec 50(12):2157-65

[46] http://www.nature.com/neuro/journal/v8/n4/full/nn1426.html

[47] Wallach, Joel D, BS, DVM, ND, Lan, Ma, MD, MS, LAc, Schrauzer, Gerhard N., PhD, MS, , FACN, CNS, *Epigenetic's: The Death Of The Genetic Theory Of Disease Transmission*, SelectBooks, Inc., New York, 2014, pp 360-361.

[48] http://www.cancer.gov/cancertopics/causes-prevention/risk/weight-activity/obesity-fact-sheet

[49] http://www.aafp.org/afp/2012/1101/p864.html

[50] http://www.drlam.com/articles/2002-No4-Andropause.asp

[51] Patrick L., Thyroid disruption: mechanism and clinical implications in human health. Altern Med Rev. 2009 December ;14 (4) :326-46.

[52] http://www.nejm.org/doi/full/10.1056/NEJMsr043743#t=article